Obesity and Gastroenterology

Editors

OCTAVIA PICKETT-BLAKELY
LINDA A. LEE

GASTROENTEROLOGY CLINICS OF NORTH AMERICA

www.gastro.theclinics.com

Consulting Editor
GARY W. FALK

December 2016 • Volume 45 • Number 4

ELSEVIER

1600 John F. Kennedy Boulevard • Suite 1800 • Philadelphia, Pennsylvania, 19103-2899
http://www.theclinics.com

GASTROENTEROLOGY CLINICS OF NORTH AMERICA Volume 45, Number 4
December 2016 ISSN 0889-8553, ISBN-13: 978-0-323-47740-6

Editor: Kerry Holland
Developmental Editor: Alison Swety

Gastroenterology Clinics of North America (ISSN 0889-8553) is published quarterly by Elsevier Inc., 360 Park Avenue South, New York, NY 10010-1710. Months of issue are March, June, September, and December. Business and Editorial Offices: 1600 John F. Kennedy Blvd., Suite 1800, Philadelphia, PA 19103-2899. Customer Service Office: 6277 Sea Harbor Drive, Orlando, FL 32887-4800. Periodicals postage paid at New York, NY and additional mailing offices. Subscription prices are $320.00 per year (US individuals), $100.00 per year (US students), $587.00 per year (US institutions), $350.00 per year (Canadian individuals), $720.00 per year (Canadian institutions), $445.00 per year (international individuals), $220.00 per year (international students), and $720.00 per year (international institutions). Foreign air speed delivery is included in all *Clinics* subscription prices. All prices are subject to change without notice. **POSTMASTER**: Send address changes to *Gastroenterology Clinics of North America*, Elsevier Health Sciences Division, Subscription Customer Service, 3251 Riverport Lane, Maryland Heights, MO 63043. **Telephone: 1-800-654-2452 (U.S. and Canada); 314-447-8871 (outside U.S. and Canada). Fax: 314-447-8029.** E-mail: **journalscustomerservice-usa@elsevier.com (for print support); journalsonlinesupport-usa@elsevier.com (for online support).**

Reprints. For copies of 100 or more, of articles in this publication, please contact the Commercial Reprints Department, Elsevier Inc., 360 Part Avenue South, New York, New York 10010-1710. Tel. 212-633-3874, Fax: 212-633-3820, E-mail: reprints@elsevier.com.

Gastroenterology Clinics of North America is also published in Italian by Il Pensiero Scientifico Editore, Rome, Italy; and in Portuguese by Interlivros Edicoes Ltda., Rua Commandante Coelho 1085, 21250 Cordovil, Rio de Janeiro, Brazil.

Gastroenterology Clinics of North America is covered in *MEDLINE/PubMed (Index Medicus), Excerpta Medica, Current Contents/Clinical Medicine, Science Citation Index, ISI/BIOMED,* and *BIOSIS*.

Contributors

CONSULTING EDITOR

GARY W. FALK, MD, MS
Professor of Medicine, Division of Gastroenterology, Hospital of the University of Pennsylvania, University of Pennsylvania Perelman School of Medicine, Philadelphia, Pennsylvania

EDITORS

OCTAVIA PICKETT-BLAKELY, MD, MHS
Assistant Professor of Medicine; Director, GI Nutrition, Obesity and Celiac Disease Program, Division of Gastroenterology, University of Pennsylvania Perelman School of Medicine, Philadelphia, Pennsylvania

LINDA A. LEE, MD
Associate Professor of Medicine; Clinical Director, Division of Gastroenterology and Hepatology, Johns Hopkins University School of Medicine; Director, Johns Hopkins Integrative Medicine and Digestive Center, Lutherville, Maryland

AUTHORS

CASSANDRA ARROYO-JOHNSON, PhD, MS
Assistant Professor, Division of Public Health Sciences, Department of Surgery, Washington University School of Medicine, St Louis, Missouri

RICARDO BADILLO, MD
Division of Gastroenterology, Washington University School of Medicine, St Louis, Missouri

MICHAEL C. BENNETT, MD
Division of Gastroenterology, Washington University School of Medicine, St Louis, Missouri

ROTONYA M. CARR, MD
Assistant Professor of Medicine, Division of Gastroenterology and Hepatology, University of Pennsylvania, Philadelphia, Pennsylvania

EUGENE B. CHANG, MD
Section of Gastroenterology, Hepatology, and Nutrition, Martin Boyer Professor of Medicine, Department of Medicine, Knapp Center for Biomedical Discovery, University of Chicago, Chicago, Illinois

DARWIN L. CONWELL, MD, MS
Section of Pancreatic Diseases, Division of Gastroenterology, Hepatology, and Nutrition, The Ohio State University Wexner Medical Center, Columbus, Ohio

ZOBEIDA CRUZ-MONSERRATE, PhD
Section of Pancreatic Diseases, Division of Gastroenterology, Hepatology, and Nutrition, The Ohio State University Wexner Medical Center; The James Comprehensive Cancer Center, The Ohio State University Wexner Medical Center, Columbus, Ohio

DANIEL T. DEMPSEY, MD
Department of Surgery, Hospital of the University of Pennsylvania, Philadelphia, Pennsylvania

KRISTOFFEL R. DUMON, MD
Department of Surgery, Hospital of the University of Pennsylvania, Philadelphia, Pennsylvania

RONALD FEINSTEIN, MD, FAAP
Professor of Pediatrics, Hofstra-Northwell School of Medicine, New Hyde Park, New York

JAMILAH GRANT-GUIMARAES, MD, FAAP
Assistant Professor of Pediatrics, Hofstra-Northwell School of Medicine, Cohen Children's Medical Center, New Hyde Park, New York

KIMBERLY GUDZUNE, MD, MPH
Assistant Professor of Medicine, Department of Medicine, Johns Hopkins University School of Medicine, Baltimore, Maryland

UMASHANKKAR KANNAN, MD
Department of Surgery, Bronx-Lebanon Hospital Center, Bronx, New York

JEANETTE N. KEITH, MD
Clinical Faculty, Alabama College of Osteopathic Medicine, Dothan, Alabama; Staff Physician, Decatur Morgan Hospital, Department of Medicine, Section of Gastroenterology; Physician, Decatur Gastroenterology Associates, P.C., Decatur, Alabama

VANDANA KHUNGAR, MD, MSc
Assistant Professor of Medicine, Division of Gastroenterology and Hepatology, University of Pennsylvania, Philadelphia, Pennsylvania

JENNIFER KOSOY, MD
Fellow, Adolescent Medicine, Cohen Children's Medical Center, New Hyde Park, New York

SOMASHEKAR G. KRISHNA, MD, MPH
Section of Pancreatic Diseases, Division of Gastroenterology, Hepatology, and Nutrition, The Ohio State University Wexner Medical Center, Columbus, Ohio

ERICA LABER, MD
Fellow, Adolescent Medicine, Cohen Children's Medical Center, New Hyde Park, New York

ELLEN E. LADENHEIM, PhD
Department of Psychiatry and Behavioral Sciences, Johns Hopkins University School of Medicine, Baltimore, Maryland

KRISTLE LEE LYNCH, MD
Assistant Professor of Medicine, Division of Gastroenterology and Hepatology,
Department of Internal Medicine, The University of Pennsylvania Health System,
Philadelphia, Pennsylvania

KRISTINA B. MARTINEZ, PhD, RD
Section of Gastroenterology, Hepatology, and Nutrition, Department of Medicine,
University of Chicago, Chicago, Illinois

KRISTA D. MINCEY, DrPH, MPH
Assistant Professor, Division of Biological and Public Health Sciences, Xavier University
of Louisiana, New Orleans, Louisiana

TIMOTHY H. MORAN, PhD
Department of Psychiatry and Behavioral Sciences, Johns Hopkins University School of
Medicine; Global Obesity Prevention Center at Johns Hopkins, Johns Hopkins
Bloomberg School of Public Health, Baltimore, Maryland

CAROLYN NEWBERRY, MD
Division of Gastroenterology, University of Pennsylvania Perelman School of Medicine,
Philadelphia, Pennsylvania

CHRISTOPHER J. NEYLAN, BA
Department of Surgery, Hospital of the University of Pennsylvania, Philadelphia,
Pennsylvania

AMANKE ORANU, MD
Division of Gastroenterology and Hepatology, University of Pennsylvania, Philadelphia,
Pennsylvania

OCTAVIA PICKETT-BLAKELY, MD, MHS
Assistant Professor of Medicine; Director, GI Nutrition, Obesity and Celiac Disease
Program, Division of Gastroenterology, University of Pennsylvania Perelman School of
Medicine, Philadelphia, Pennsylvania

JOSEPH F. PIERRE, PhD
Section of Gastroenterology, Hepatology, and Nutrition, Department of Medicine,
University of Chicago, Chicago, Illinois

SHELBY SULLIVAN, MD
Division of Gastroenterology, University of Colorado School of Medicine, Aurora,
Colorado

NOEL N. WILLIAMS, MD
Department of Surgery, Hospital of the University of Pennsylvania, Philadelphia,
Pennsylvania

Contents

mortality of esophageal adenocarcinoma, identification of risk factors for Barrett's esophagus and esophageal adenocarcinoma is crucial. There are a plethora of studies investigating the relationship of obesity with these pathologies. Recent studies reveal that this relationship may specifically be with central adiposity. Increased cell turnover and eventual carcinogenesis is likely precipitated by increased intragastric pressure but also is affected by the complex interplay of increased insulin resistance in patients with increased fat tissue. Further studies are warranted to evaluate if weight loss can decrease progression of Barrett's esophagus.

Obesity is a well-recognized risk factor for gallstone formation and increases the risk for gallstone-related complications. Pancreatic diseases are impacted adversely by obesity. Although weight loss surgery increases the risk of gallstone disease, evidence suggests that bariatric surgery mitigates the obesity-associated adverse prognostication in acute pancreatitis. Obesity is also a significant risk factor for pancreatic cancer. Obesity is a global epidemic and is increasing worldwide and among all age groups. There is an urgent need for focused health policies aimed at reducing the incidence and prevalence of obesity. This article summarizes the current literature highlighting the association between obesity and the pathophysiology and outcome of gallstone disease, pancreatitis, and pancreatic cancer.

Nonalcoholic fatty liver disease (NAFLD) is an important cause of morbidity and mortality worldwide and is rapidly becoming the leading cause of end-stage liver disease and liver transplant. With a prevalence of 30% in the United States, it has reached epidemic proportions. The clinical syndrome of NAFLD spans from bland steatosis to steatohepatitis, which can progress to fibrosis and cirrhosis. The pathogenesis includes the roles of hormones, nutritional and intestinal dysbiosis, insulin resistance, lipotoxicity, hepatic inflammation, and genes. Noninvasive testing and liver biopsy indications are reviewed. Approved and investigational therapies for NAFLD and nonalcoholic steatohepatitis are outlined in this article.

Given the prevalence of overweight and obesity and their associated health conditions, clinicians will be increasingly tasked with the responsibility of addressing overweight and obesity. This article reviews the 5As approach—assess, advise, agree, assist, arrange—and how clinicians can use the approach facilitate weight management discussions with their patients that met the recommendations provided in the 2013 adult weight management guidelines issued by the American Heart Association/American College of Cardiology/The Obesity Society.

Common disease states in gastroenterology are more effectively treated in an obese patient when weight loss is incorporated into the treatment plan. Strategies that seek to achieve weight loss improve outcomes in the treatment of hepatitis C, non-alcoholic fatty liver disease, and colorectal cancer, as examples. Pharmacologic therapy is an important adjunctive intervention that improves both short-term and long-term outcomes in the management of obese patients. This article reviews currently available drug therapy with a focus on pharmacotherapy approved long-term weight management in non-diabetic obese individuals since 2012, encouraging the use of these tools in the practice of gastroenterology.

Endoscopic bariatric therapy consists of devices or procedures for primary weight loss or weight regain after Roux-en-Y gastric bypass that are placed or done endoscopically. In most cases, they result in less weight loss, but fewer complications than bariatric surgery; and more weight loss than lifestyle therapy or weight loss medications. These therapies are important advances to treat patients with obesity. This article focuses on therapies or devices with US Food and Drug Administration approval or those with current or planned US pivotal trials.

In the United States, more than one-third of the population is obese. Currently, bariatric surgery is the best known treatment for obesity, and multiple meta-analyses have shown bariatric surgery to be more effective for treating obesity than diet and exercise or pharmacologic treatment. The modern era of bariatric surgery began in 2005, which is defined by a drastic increase in the use of laparoscopy. Bariatric surgery has the potential to improve obesity-related comorbidities, such as type 2 diabetes, cardiovascular disease, and sleep apnea. The effect of bariatric surgery on weight loss and comorbidities varies by the type of procedure.

Although diet and exercise have been the cornerstone of therapy for obesity, efficacy is suboptimal and short lived. Surgical procedures are durable but invasive therapy for obesity. Supplemental therapies for obesity that are minimally invasive, low risk, and effective are needed. Several therapeutic options are being developed that offer obese patients and their health care providers alternatives to what is currently available.

Childhood overweight and obesity are increasing in prevalence and are a growing health concern. The diseases and their comorbidities have devastating consequences to children and adults as well as families, communities, and the nation. Comorbidities are cardiorespiratory, endocrinologic, gastrointestinal, orthopedic, and psychosocial. Health care providers are facing this crisis with limited medical, community, and federal resources and insufficient reimbursement. This article reviews recent trends in the assessment and treatment of this disease as well as trends in reimbursement, financial implications, and the need for further research and advocacy.

GASTROENTEROLOGY
CLINICS OF NORTH AMERICA

THE CLINICS ARE AVAILABLE ONLINE!
Access your subscription at:
www.theclinics.com

Preface

Obesity and Gastroenterology

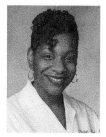 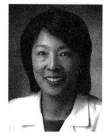

Octavia Pickett-Blakely, MD, MHS   Linda A. Lee, MD
Editors

Overweight and obesity have emerged as major threats to public health all over the world. The 2013 Burden of Disease Study demonstrated that the worldwide proportion of women with a body mass index >25 grew from 30% in 1980 to 38% in 2013, while for men the proportion grew from 29 to 37% during the same time period.[1] In the United States, overweight and obesity have reached epidemic proportions in 2015 with nearly 70% of adults and 30% of children having a body mass index that falls into one of these categories. Although countries associated with high income have historically had the highest prevalence, the prevalence of overweight and obesity is rising in countries of low and middle incomes. Given the far-reaching effects of obesity on health and disease, understanding the causes, consequences, and best management approaches is critical in all fields of medicine today.

This issue of *Gastroenterology Clinics of North America* illustrates the growing complexity of obesity by reviewing the physiology and behavioral and socioeconomic issues that contribute to its pathogenesis while placing emphasis on gastrointestinal and liver diseases. The latest therapies are included, covering a spectrum of behavioral approaches, pharmacologic interventions, endoscopic and surgical procedures, and manipulation of the gut microbiota to optimize metabolism and energy utilization. The treatment of overweight and obesity should be integrated into any therapeutic strategy when dealing with common chronic gastrointestinal and liver disorders, including gastroesophageal reflux, gallstones, fatty liver disease, and pancreatic disease. Practical advice is provided in these articles by experts to help those interested

Gastroenterol Clin N Am 45 (2016) xiii–xiv
http://dx.doi.org/10.1016/j.gtc.2016.09.001
0889-8553/16/© 2016 Published by Elsevier Inc.

in utilizing evidence-based dietary, behavioral pharmacologic, and surgical approaches, or wishing to overcome the obstacles of managing childhood obesity.

Octavia Pickett-Blakely, MD, MHS
Assistant Professor of Medicine
Director, GI Nutrition, Obesity and Celiac Disease Program
Division of Gastroenterology
University of Pennsylvania
Perelman School of Medicine
3400 Civic Center Boulevard
4 South
Philadelphia, PA 19104, USA

Linda A. Lee, MD
Associate Professor of Medicine
Clinical Director, Division of Gastroenterology and Hepatology
Johns Hopkins University School of Medicine
Director, Johns Hopkins Integrative Medicine
and Digestive Center
2360 West Joppa Road, Suite 200
Lutherville, MD 21093, USA

E-mail addresses:
octavia.pickett-blakely@uphs.upenn.edu (O. Pickett-Blakely)
llee12@jhmi.edu (L.A. Lee)

REFERENCE

1. Ng M, Fleming T, Robinson M, et al. Global, regional, and national prevalence of overweight and obesity in children and adults during 1980-2013: a systematic analysis for the Global Burden of Disease Study 2013. Lancet 2014;384:766–81.

Obesity Epidemiology Worldwide

Cassandra Arroyo-Johnson, PhD, MS[a],*, Krista D. Mincey, DrPH, MPH[b]

KEYWORDS

- Obesity • Epidemiology • BMI • Racial/ethnic disparities
- Social determinants of health

KEY POINTS

- Trends in obesity prevalence over the past 2 decades have increased across the globe while remaining high in the United States.
- Obesity, for screening purposes, is defined as a body mass index (BMI) greater than or equal to 30 kg/m^2 for adults and BMI above the age- and sex-specific 95th percentile of the Centers for Disease Control and Prevention or World Health Organization growth charts.
- Obesity is higher among women, racial/ethnic groups, and at lower levels of education and income.
- Data collection of ethnic subgroups across all races will improve the ability to monitor trends in obesity and potential other health outcomes over time.
- It is critical to consider both individual behaviors and social determinants of health for identifying at-risk populations to develop evidence-based, culturally relevant clinical and population interventions.

INTRODUCTION

Obesity continues to be a public health concern across the globe. Obesity has a demonstrated association with health behaviors[1–8] and health outcomes, such as diabetes, hypertension, and cancer.[9–14] Over the past 2 decades, obesity has increased worldwide and remains highest in the United States. It is critical to understand the definition of obesity, using body mass index (BMI) appropriately, recent estimates, and

The authors have no conflicts of interests to disclose; this article was supported by the National Cancer Institute (U54CA155496), the Foundation for Barnes-Jewish Hospital, Alvin J. Siteman Cancer Center, and Washington University School of Medicine Department of Surgery.
a Division of Public Health Sciences, Department of Surgery, Washington University School of Medicine, 660 South Euclid Avenue, Campus Box 8100, St Louis, MO 63110, USA; b Division of Biological and Public Health Sciences, Xavier University of Louisiana, 1 Drexel Drive, Campus Box V, New Orleans, LA 70125, USA
* Corresponding author.
E-mail address: johnsonca@wudosis.wustl.edu

Gastroenterol Clin N Am 45 (2016) 571–579
http://dx.doi.org/10.1016/j.gtc.2016.07.012
0889-8553/16/© 2016 Elsevier Inc. All rights reserved.

gastro.theclinics.com

risk factors as a framework within which clinicians should work to help reduce the burden of obesity and obesity-related health outcomes. This framework, including the Healthy People 2020 place-based approach to social determinants of health, is described in this article.

DEFINITION AND MEASUREMENT

BMI is the most common measure used for population and clinical screening for obesity. Weight and height are needed for BMI and usually determined using measured weight and height in clinical settings and self-reported weight and height in larger population health studies. BMI is calculated as one's weight in kilograms divided by one's height in meters squared (kg/m^2). Although the definition of obesity is dependent on the method used to determine the presence of obesity (ie, BMI, waist circumference), for the purpose of this article, obesity is defined based on the World Health Organization's international adult classification of BMI (**Table 1**).

Currently, there is no consensus on an international classification of BMI for children. However, for the purpose of this article, obesity is classified as BMI greater than or equal to the age- and sex-specific 95th percentile based on the 2000 Centers for Disease Control and Prevention growth charts.[15]

OBESITY WORLDWIDE

- Over the past 3 and half decades, the prevalence of obesity has nearly doubled worldwide.[16]
- Among adults aged 18 years or older, 11% of men and 15% of women were obese in 2014.
- More than 42 million children under the age of 5 years were overweight in 2013.

Table 1
International classification of adult underweight, overweight, and obesity according to body mass index

Classification	BMI (kg/m^2) Principal Cutoff Points	BMI (kg/m^2) Additional Cutoff Points
Underweight	<18.50	<18.50
Severe thinness	<16.00	<16.00
Moderate thinness	16.00–16.99	16.00–16.99
Mild thinness	17.00–18.49	17.00–18.49
Normal range	18.50–24.99	18.50–22.99 23.00–24.99
Overweight	≥25.00	≥25.00
Preobese	25.00–29.99	25.00–27.49 27.50–29.99
Obese	≥30.00	≥30.00
Obese class I	30.00–34.99	30.00–32.49 32.50–34.99
Obese class II	35.00–39.99	35.00–37.49 37.50–39.99
Obese class III	≥40.00	≥40.00

From World Health Organization. BMI Classification. 2016.

OBESITY IN NORTH AMERICA

- In the United States, the prevalence of obesity among adults over the age of 20 is approximately 36%.[17]
- 38.3% of women and 34.3% of men in the United States are obese, and obesity prevalence in the United States varies by gender (**Fig. 1**), race/ethnicity (**Fig. 2**), and socioeconomic status.[17]
- Canada has lower adult obesity prevalence than the United States across gender (**Fig. 3**).[18]
- Among children, the prevalence of obesity in the United States was 17% in 2011 to 2014, and similar to adults, prevalence also varies by gender, age (**Fig. 4**), and race/ethnicity (**Fig. 5**).[17]
- Canada also has lower childhood and adolescent obesity prevalence than the United States across gender (**Fig. 6**).[19]

Special consideration needs to be given to ethnic subgroups among Hispanics because there are cultural differences that may impact obesity in different ways. The Hispanic prevalence of obesity based on the National Health and Nutrition Examination Survey estimates provided above are based on a sample of Mexican and Mexican Americans, the largest Hispanic subgroup in the United States.[20] Studies have shown that there are ethnic variations in obesity, behaviors, risk factors, demographics, and social determinants among Hispanics.[21–27] These variations become masked in a pan-ethnic grouping and may impact both clinical and population interventions for obesity reduction and prevention targeted toward Hispanics in the United States.[21–26,28–30]

OBESITY RISK FACTORS

- Energy imbalance between nutrition and physical activity[31–34]
- Direct and indirect genetic effects[35,36]

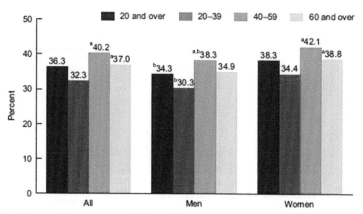

Fig. 1. Obesity prevalence among adults aged 20 and over, by sex and age: National Health and Nutrition Examination Survey, 2011 to 2014. [a] Significantly different from those aged 20 to 39. [b] Significantly different from women of the same age group. NOTE: Totals were age adjusted by the direct method to the 2000 US census population using the age groups 20 to 39, 40 to 59, and 60 and over. Crude estimates are 36.5% for all, 34.5% for men, and 38.5% for women. (*From* Ogden CL, Carroll MD, Fryar CD, et al. Prevalence of obesity among adults and youth: United States, 2011–2014. NCHS Data Brief 2015;219.)

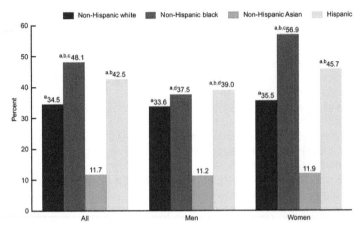

Fig. 2. Obesity prevalence among adults aged 20 and over, by sex and race and Hispanic origin: United States, 2011 to 2014. [a] Significantly different from non-Hispanic Asian persons. [b] Significantly different from non-Hispanic white persons. [c] Significantly different from Hispanic persons. [d] Significantly different from women of the same race and Hispanic origin. NOTE: All estimates are age adjusted by the direct method to the 2000 US census population using the age groups 20 to 39, 40 to 59, and 60 and over. (*From* Ogden CL, Carroll MD, Fryar CD, et al. Prevalence of obesity among adults and youth: United States, 2011–2014. NCHS Data Brief 2015;219.)

- Gene-environment interactions[37]
- Social determinants of health (**Fig. 7**)[38]

Social determinants of health are defined as the contexts of the environments in which people are born, live, learn, work, play, worship, and age that affect a wide range of health, functioning, and quality-of-life outcomes and risks.[38] In the context

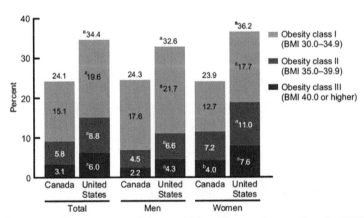

Fig. 3. Obesity prevalence among adults aged 20 to 79 years, by sex: Canada, 2007 to 2009 and United States, 2007 to 2008. [a] Statistically different from estimate for Canada (*P*<.05). [b] Use with caution (coefficient of variation 16.6%–33.3%). NOTE: Estimates were age standardized by the direct method to the 2000 US Census population using age groups 20 to 39, 40 to 59, and 60 to 79. Pregnant women are excluded. Obesity class estimates do not sum to exact totals due to rounding. (*From* Shields M, Carroll MD, Ogden CL. Adult obesity prevalence in Canada and the United States. NCHS Data Brief 2011;56.)

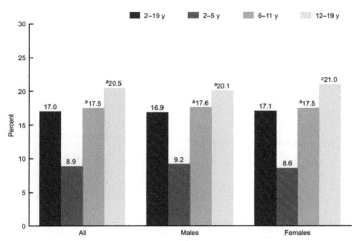

Fig. 4. Obesity prevalence among youth aged 2 to 19 years, by sex and age: National Health and Nutrition Examination Survey, 2011 to 2014. [a] Significantly different from those aged 2 to 5 years. (*From* Ogden CL, Carroll MD, Fryar CD, et al. Prevalence of obesity among adults and youth: United States, 2011–2014. NCHS Data Brief 2015;219.)

of that complex environment, social determinants of health include physical and social determinants. Examples of physical determinants of obesity include the following[38]:

- Green spaces and other natural elements of the environment
- Parks, buildings, sidewalks, bike lanes, and other aspects of the built environment[39]

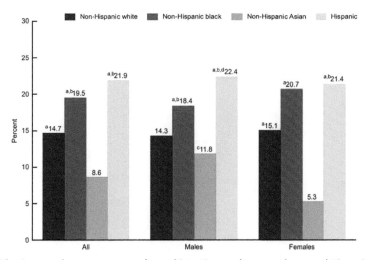

Fig. 5. Obesity prevalence among youth aged 2 to 19 years, by sex and race and Hispanic origin: National Health and Nutrition Examination Survey, 2011 to 2014. [a] Significantly different from non-Hispanic Asians. [b] Significantly different from non-Hispanic whites. [c] Significantly different from girls of the same race and Hispanic origin. [d] Significantly different from non-Hispanic blacks. (*From* Ogden CL, Carroll MD, Fryar CD, et al. Prevalence of obesity among adults and youth: United States, 2011–2014. NCHS Data Brief 2015;219.)

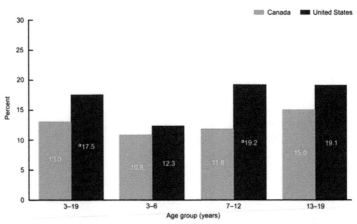

Fig. 6. Obesity prevalence among children and adolescents aged 3 to 19 years, by sex: Canada, 2009 to 2013, and United States, 2009 to 2012. [a] Statistically significant difference compared with Canada ($P<.05$). NOTE: Pregnant girls are excluded. (*From* Carroll MD, Navaneelan T, Bryan S, et al. Prevalence of obesity among children and adolescents in the United States and Canada. NCHS Data Brief 2015;211.)

- Schools, recreation facilities and programs, and work sites
- Physical barriers limiting people with disabilities

Some examples of social determinants of obesity include the following[38]:

- Socioeconomic conditions (ie, concentrated poverty)
- Residential segregation

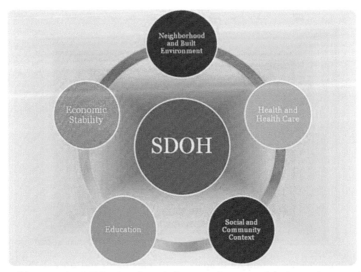

Fig. 7. Healthy People 2020 place-based framework on social determinants of health. SDOH, Social Determinants of Health. (*From* Office of Disease Prevention and Health Promotion. Social Determinants of Health. Heal People 2020. 2014. Available at: https://www.healthypeople.gov/2020/topics-objectives/topic/social-determinants-of-health. Accessed July 7, 2016.)

- Access to health care services
- Transportation options
- Availability of resources to meet daily needs
- Social support

For clinicians, patient obesity management and reduction instructions and programs should also take into account social determinants, which could serve to improve patient capacity to make necessary behavioral changes. Clinicians, patients, and public health professionals should actively work together and may use epidemiologic evidence linking obesity to social determinants to advocate for policy-level interventions as well.

SUMMARY

Obesity is a global public health concern, with the highest rates found in the United States. Although obesity prevalence worldwide varies at the national level, there are also significant differences across gender, socioeconomic status, and race/ethnicity, particularly in the United States, where obesity is highest. Future clinical research should include capturing clinical data for more precise estimation of national, regional, and local trends over time by race/ethnicity and education to calculate estimates of obesity prevalence worldwide. Racial and ethnic variations in adult and youth obesity also require further research.[21] For example, although the specific mechanisms by which education impacts obesity prevalence at the national level need further exploration, policy to improve high school graduation rates, college enrollment, retention, and graduation can benefit all racial and ethnic groups. In addition, there is an urgent need to evaluate the effectiveness of obesity interventions for prevention and control.[16] Finally, clinicians should consider using epidemiologic evidence linking obesity to social determinants to advocate for policy-level interventions to improve social and physical environment conditions for obesity prevention and intervention.

REFERENCES

1. Quick VM, McWilliams R, Byrd-Bredbenner C. Fatty, fatty, two-by-four: weight-teasing history and disturbed eating in young adult women. Am J Public Health 2013;103(3):508–15.

2. Wang H, Steffen LM, Zhou X, et al. Consistency between increasing trends in added-sugar intake and body mass index among adults: the Minnesota Heart Survey, 1980-1982 to 2007-2009. Am J Public Health 2013;103(3):501–7.

3. Block JP, Scribner RA, DeSalvo KB. Fast food, race/ethnicity, and income: a geographic analysis. Am J Prev Med 2004;27(3):211–7.

4. Boardman JD, Saint Onge JM, Rogers RG, et al. Race differential in obesity: the impact of place. J Health Soc Behav 2005;46(3):229–43.

5. Drewnowski A, Specter SE. Poverty and obesity: the role of energy density and energy costs. Am J Clin Nutr 2004;79(1):6–16. Available at: http://www.ncbi.nlm.nih.gov/pubmed/14684391.

6. Gibson DM. The neighborhood food environment and adult weight status: estimates from longitudinal data. Am J Public Health 2011;101(1):71–8.

7. Abell JE, Egan BM, Wilson PWF, et al. Age and race impact the association between BMI and CVD mortality in women. Public Health Rep 2007;122(4):507–12. Available at: http://www.pubmedcentral.nih.gov/articlerender.fcgi?artid=1888501&tool=pmcentrez&rendertype=abstract.

8. Corral I, Landrine H, Hao Y, et al. Residential segregation, health behavior and overweight/obesity among a national sample of African American adults. J Health Psychol 2012;17(3):371–8.

9. Zhang H, Rodriguez-Monguio R. Racial disparities in the risk of developing obesity-related diseases: a cross-sectional study. Ethn Dis 2012;22(3):308–16.

10. Dehal A, Garrett T, Tedders SH, et al. Body mass index and death rate of colorectal cancer among a national cohort of U.S. adults. Nutr Cancer 2011;63(8):1218–25.

11. Vranian M, Blaha M, Silverman M, et al. The interaction of fitness, fatness, and cardiometabolic risk. J Am Coll Cardiol 2012;59(13):E1754.

12. Willey JZ, Rodriguez CJ, Carlino RF, et al. Race-ethnic differences in the association between lipid profile components and risk of myocardial infarction: the Northern Manhattan Study. Am Heart J 2011;161(5):886–92.

13. Ma Y, Hébert JR, Manson JE, et al. Determinants of racial/ethnic disparities in incidence of diabetes in postmenopausal women in the U.S.: the Women's Health Initiative 1993-2009. Diabetes Care 2012;35(11):2226–34.

14. Liu X, Liu M, Tsilimingras D, et al. Racial disparities in cardiovascular risk factors among diagnosed hypertensive subjects. J Am Soc Hypertens 2011;5(4):239–48.

15. Kuczmarski RJ, Ogden CL, Guo SS, et al. 2000 CDC growth charts for the United States: methods and development. Vital Health Stat 11 2002;246:1–190.

16. World Health Organization (WHO). Global Status Report on Noncommunicable Diseases 2014. Switzerland: WHO; 2014.

17. Ogden CL, Carroll MD, Fryar CD, et al. Prevalence of Obesity among Adults and Youth: United States, 2011-2014. Hyattsville (MD): National Center for Health Statistics; 2015.

18. Shields M, Carroll MD, Ogden CL. Adult Obesity Prevalence in Canada and the United States Are There Differences in Obesity Prevalence Estimates between Canada and the United States? Key Findings. Hyattsville (MD): National Center for Health Statistics; 2007.

19. Carroll MD, Navaneelan T, Bryan S, et al. Prevalence of Obesity among Children and Adolescents in the United States and Canada. Hyattsville (MD): National Center for Health Statistics; 2015.

20. Ogden CL, Carroll MD, Kit BK, et al. Prevalence of childhood and adult obesity in the United States, 2011-2012. JAMA 2014;311(8):806–14.

21. Arroyo-Johnson C, Mincey KD, Ackermann N, et al. Racial and ethnic heterogeneity in self-reported diabetes prevalence trends across Hispanic subgroups, National Health Interview Survey, 1997-2012. Prev Chronic Dis 2016;13(E10):1–10.

22. Borrell LN. Racial identity among Hispanics: implications for health and well-being. Am J Public Health 2005;95(3):379–81.

23. Borrell LN, Crawford ND. Disparities in self-reported hypertension in Hispanic subgroups, non-Hispanic black and non-Hispanic white adults: the National Health Interview survey. Ann Epidemiol 2008;18(10):803–12.

24. Borrell LN, Crawford ND, Dallo FJ, et al. Self-reported diabetes in Hispanic subgroup, non-Hispanic black, and non-Hispanic white populations: National Health Interview Survey, 1997-2005. Public Health Rep 2009;124(5):702–10. Available at: http://www.pubmedcentral.nih.gov/articlerender.fcgi?artid=2728662&tool=pmcentrez&rendertype=abstract.

25. Borrell LN, Crawford ND. All-cause mortality among Hispanics in the United States: exploring heterogeneity by nativity status, country of origin, and race in

the National Health Interview Survey-linked mortality files. Ann Epidemiol 2009; 19(5):336–43.

26. Borrell LN, Lancet EA. Race/ethnicity and all-cause mortality in US adults: revisiting the Hispanic paradox. Am J Public Health 2012;102(5):836–43.

27. Crespo CJ, Loria CM, Burt VL. Hypertension and other cardiovascular disease risk factors among Mexican Americans, Cuban Americans, and Puerto Ricans from the Hispanic Health and Nutrition Examination Survey. Public Health Rep 1996; 111(Suppl 2):7–10. Available at: http://www.pubmedcentral.nih.gov/articlerender. fcgi?artid=1381652&tool=pmcentrez&rendertype=abstract.

28. Martinez-Tyson D, Pathak EB, Soler-Vila H, et al. Looking under the Hispanic umbrella: cancer mortality among Cubans, Mexicans, Puerto Ricans and other Hispanics in Florida. J Immigr Minor Health 2009;11(4):249–57.

29. Pinheiro PS, Williams M, Miller EA, et al. Cancer survival among Latinos and the Hispanic paradox. Cancer Causes Control 2011;22(4):553–61.

30. Daviglus ML, Talavera G a, Avilés-Santa ML, et al. Prevalence of major cardiovascular risk factors and cardiovascular diseases among Hispanic/Latino individuals of diverse backgrounds in the United States. J Am Med Assoc 2012;308(17): 1775–84.

31. Sallis JF, Glanz K. Physical activity and food environments: solutions to the obesity epidemic. Milbank Q 2009;87(1):123–54.

32. Flegal KM, Carroll MD, Kuczmarski RJ, et al. Obesity and related health behaviors among urban and rural children in the United States: data from the National Health And Nutrition Examination Survey 2003-2004 and 2005-2006. JAMA 2014; 311(1):806–14.

33. Clark BR, White ML, Royer NK, et al. Obesity and aerobic fitness among urban public school students in elementary, middle, and high school. Ciccozzi M, ed. PLoS One 2015;10(9):e0138175.

34. Mobley LR, Root ED, Finkelstein EA, et al. Environment, obesity, and cardiovascular disease risk in low-income women. Am J Prev Med 2006;30(4):327–32.

35. Johnson RJ, Stenvinkel P, Martin SL, et al. Redefining metabolic syndrome as a fat storage condition based on studies of comparative physiology. Obesity (Silver Spring) 2013;21(4):659–64.

36. Speakman JR. Functional analysis of seven genes linked to body mass index and adiposity by genome-wide association studies: a review. Hum Hered 2013; 75(2–4):57–79.

37. Phelan JC, Link BG. Controlling disease and creating disparities: a fundamental cause perspective. J Gerontol B Psychol Sci Soc Sci 2005;60(Spec No 2):27–33.

38. Office of Disease Prevention and Health Promotion. Social Determinants of Health. Heal People 2020. 2014. Available at: https://www.healthypeople.gov/ 2020/topics-objectives/topic/social-determinants-of-health. Accessed July 7, 2016.

39. Arroyo-Johnson C, Woodward K, Milam L, et al. Still separate, still unequal: Social determinants of playground safety and proximity. J Urban Health 2016;93: 627–38.

Physiologic and Neural Controls of Eating

Timothy H. Moran, PhD[a,b,*], Ellen E. Ladenheim, PhD[a]

KEYWORDS

- Nutrient availability • Adiposity signaling • Satiety signals • Reward processing
- Eating

KEY POINTS

- Multiple physiologic and neural systems contribute to the controls over what and how much we eat.
- These systems include signaling involved in the detection and signaling of nutrient availability, signals arising from consumed nutrients that provide feedback information during a meal to induce satiation, and signals related to the rewarding properties of eating.
- Each of these has a separate neural representation but important interactions among these systems are critical to the overall controls of food intake.

What and how much we choose to eat are influenced by a variety of factors. These include the palatability or taste of particular foods, what we have learned about specific foods through experience, social and cultural influences on what foods and what amounts of food are appropriate to consume, the relative availability and the cost of specific foods, and an interacting system of physiologic controls that serve to both maintain adequate nutrition and limit intake to maximize our use of consumed nutrients. The recent obesity epidemic makes it clear that environmental influences can have a tremendous effect on overall energy balance. Obesity rates began to increase in the United States in the 1970s and this can all be attributed to changes in the food environment. However, the changing food environment interacts with a set of physiologic controls that are important in the meal-to-meal controls of eating.

In this review, we concentrate on the roles of 3 interacting physiologic and neural systems important in feeding control (**Fig. 1**). These are systems that mediate (1) signals related to metabolic state and nutrient availability, (2) signals that arise during a

Disclosures: T.H. Moran is a consultant for Healthways and Novo Nordisk. E.E. Ladenheim has nothing to declare.
[a] Department of Psychiatry and Behavioral Sciences, Johns Hopkins University School of Medicine, 720 Rutland Avenue, Baltimore, MD 21205, USA; [b] Global Obesity Prevention Center at Johns Hopkins, Johns Hopkins Bloomberg School of Public Health, 615 N. Wolfe Street, Baltimore, MD 21205, USA
* Corresponding author. Department of Psychiatry and Behavioral Sciences, Johns Hopkins University School of Medicine, Ross 618, 720 Rutland Avenue, Baltimore, MD 21205.
E-mail address: tmoran@jhmi.edu

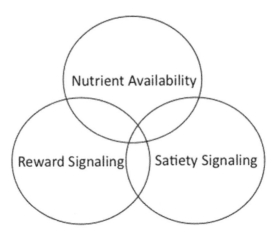

Fig. 1. Overall physiologic controls of eating behavior.

meal that serve to end that meal and maintain as state of satiety, and (3) affective signals related to taste and nutritional consequences that serve to reinforce aspects of eating. We will also identify how these systems interact in the defense of overall energy balance.

NUTRIENT AVAILABILITY SIGNALING

Studies of rodent genetic obesity models had long suggested the importance of circulating factors in overall body weight control. Having identified 2 different mutations in mice that led to obesity,[1] led to parabiosis experiments involving 2 strains of obese (obese [ob/ob] and diabetic [db/db]) and normal mice in which the blood supply between 2 mice in a parabiotic pair was shared. The results led to the conclusion that ob/ob mice lacked a circulating satiety factor that, in its absence, results in greatly increased food intake and obesity, whereas the db/db mouse produced the factor but lacked the ability to appropriately respond to that factor. Twenty years later, Friedman and colleagues[2] cloned the ob gene and named the protein that it produced "leptin" from the Greek "leptos" meaning thin, because this was a factor that helped maintain a normal body weight. Shortly thereafter, the leptin receptor protein was identified as the product of the db gene.[3,4] Leptin is produced primarily in white fat and circulating leptin levels correlate positively with the fat mass, increasing in circulation as animals or humans become obese.[5] Thus, leptin serves as a signal of the available stored energy.

The study of leptin's actions has illuminated many of the brain circuits that contribute critically to the control of energy balance and provided a basis for understanding earlier lesion work demonstrating a role for hypothalamic nuclei in energy balance. Leptin receptors are expressed throughout the brain with a particularly high expression within hypothalamic nuclei and other brain regions with identified roles in energy balance.[6] Interactions of leptin with its receptors within these hypothalamic nuclei result in the activation or inactivation of hypothalamic pathways containing various peptides that when administered into the brain either stimulate or stop eating.[7,8]

A major hypothalamic site of leptin's actions is the arcuate nucleus. The arcuate contains 2 distinct neuronal populations that express leptin receptors. The first are neurons that express the prepropeptide proopiomelanocortin (POMC). POMC is processed into multiple opioid and melanocortin peptides including the anorexigenic peptide α-melanocyte stimulating hormone. Central administration of α-melanocyte stimulating hormone or synthetic melanocortin agonists potently inhibits food intake.[9,10] Leptin activates POMC neurons,[11] resulting in both increased POMC expression[12] and α-melanocyte stimulating hormone release at terminal sites.[13] Arcuate nucleus POMC expression decreases with food deprivation[14] and increases with overfeeding,[15] suggesting a regulatory role for this peptide in overall feeding control. Important roles for melanocortin signaling in energy balance have been demonstrated in experiments examining the effects of POMC[16] and melanocortin-3 or melanocortin-4 receptor[17] knockouts. Furthermore, genetic mutations in various aspects of the melanocortin signaling pathway have been identified as monogenic causes of human obesity.[18]

Leptin also interacts with arcuate neurons that express the orexigenic peptides, neuropeptide Y (NPY) and the endogenous melanocortin antagonist agouti-related peptide (AgRP). Leptin inhibits neuronal activity in these cells, reducing NPY and AgRP release[13] and downregulates the expression of these peptides.[7] When leptin levels are low, in times of nutrient depletion or food restriction, the leptin inhibitory tone on NPY/AgRP neurons is diminished, activity in these neurons is increased, and the orexigenic peptides NPY and AgRP are released. Lesions of these NPY/AgRP–containing neurons in adulthood results in rapid starvation.[19]

The feeding stimulatory actions of both NPY and AgRP have been well-documented. Intracerebroventricular or direct hypothalamic injection of NPY potently stimulates feeding[20–23] and repeated or chronic NPY administration results in obesity. Cell bodies of neurons expressing NPY are found in multiple hypothalamic nuclei, including the arcuate and dorsomedial hypothalamic nuclei.[24] Chronic treatment with NPY or viral-induced NPY overexpression[25,26] can result in obesity.

AgRP is an endogenous melanocortin antagonist whose expression is limited to the NPY/AgRP–expressing neurons within the arcuate nucleus. AgRP expression is upregulated in response to fasting.[27] AgRP or synthetic melanocortin antagonists increase food intake when administered into the brain and their effects are long lasting.[9,28] GABAergic signaling is an additional important output of NPY/AgRP expressing neurons in their interactions with arcuate POMC neurons exerting an inhibitory tone on anorexigenic signaling[11] and on neurons in the midbrain parabrachial nucleus.[29]

The hypothalamic paraventricular nucleus and the perifornical area of the lateral hypothalamus are important projection sites for arcuate POMC and NPY/AgRP neurons. The paraventricular nucleus contains neuronal populations that mainly express anorexigenic peptides and thus the outputs from this nucleus serve to limit food intake. Leptin and/or melanocortins activate paraventricular nucleus neurons containing corticotrophin releasing factor,[30–32] oxytocin,[33] and gastrin-releasing peptide[34] and each of these peptides reduce food intake when centrally administered.[35–37]

The perifornical region of the lateral hypothalamus contains neurons expressing the orexigenic peptides orexin and melanin concentrating hormone (MCH). Preproorexin expression is increased in response to deprivation and decreased in response to leptin administration[38] and central orexin administration increases food intake.[39] Furthermore, administration of an orexin 1 receptor antagonist inhibits eating, suggesting a role for endogenous orexin in food intake control.[40] MCH expressing cells are located similarly in the perifornical region of the lateral hypothalamus, although they represent a distinct neuronal population. MCH expression is increased in response to fasting[41] and is decreased by leptin administration.[42] MCH administration increases food intake in a dose-related fashion[43] and genetic overexpression of MCH results in obesity.[44]

Although leptin is the adiposity signal that has received the most attention, insulin also acts in the hypothalamus as an adiposity signal. Insulin levels increase with increased adiposity, insulin is transported from the circulation into the brain, and insulin receptors are localized to the hypothalamus with a high concentration in the arcuate nucleus.[45] Central insulin administration inhibits food intake[46] and has been shown to modulate activity in the leptin responsive arcuate circuit, decreasing NPY messenger RNA expression[47] and increasing activity in POMC neurons.[48]

Arcuate neurons that respond to leptin and insulin have also been proposed to be responsive to alterations in the local concentrations of nutrients and in this way serve as sensors for both short- and long-term nutrient states.[49] For example, arcuate POMC neurons are activated[50] and NPY/AgRP expressing neurons can be either activated or inhibited by increasing glucose concentration.[51] However, the role of these glucose-induced alterations in electrophysiologic activity in the control of eating is uncertain as brain glucose concentrations do not necessarily reflect changes in circulating glucose or increase in response to meals.[52] Hypothalamic neurons are also responsive to changes in the local concentration of fatty acids[53,54] and intraventricular administration of a long chain fatty acid has been shown to reduce food intake.[55] These data have been interpreted to suggest a role for brain fatty acid concentrations as signaling nutrient availability.[56] Finally, local hypothalamic administration of some amino acids has been shown to decrease food intake.[57,58] However, whether such a mechanism is involved in signaling circulating protein availability has yet to be demonstrated.

Although the hypothalamus has been a primary focus of the study of anorexigenic and orexigenic neuropeptide signaling, the neural pathways regulating energy balance are clearly distributed to multiple brain sites. For example, leptin receptors are expressed in the nucleus of the solitary tract (NTS) in the dorsal hindbrain.[59] Local leptin administration at this site reduces food intake and downregulation of NTS leptin receptors attenuates the ability of leptin to reduce food intake.[60,61] Data such as these strongly support the view that the adiposity controls of food intake are distributed rather than simply localized to the hypothalamic arcuate nucleus.[62,63]

SATIETY SIGNALING

In people and many experimental models for the study of feeding control, eating is not a continuous activity, but occurs in distinct bouts or meals. Meal initiation is determined by a variety of factors, especially food availability. During a meal, ingested nutrients contact a variety of receptors within the oral cavity and gastrointestinal tract resulting in neural and hormonal signals that contribute to the determination of meal size. Meal size can be highly variable and alterations in meal size seem to be a major determinant of overall food intake.

Taste plays a major role in both food choice and in the amount of a particular food that is consumed. The effects of taste on overall ingestion are best demonstrated under conditions in which the feedback from the gastrointestinal tract is minimized. Experimental paradigms that specifically assess the effects of taste or palatability on ingestion have been commonly used. The first of these is called "sham feeding," in which animals have an esophageal or gastric fistula so that consumed liquid nutrients drain out of the fistula and do not accumulate in the stomach or pass on to the intestine. Such a preparation was first used by Pavlov.[64] Pavlov demonstrated that dogs with open esophageal fistulas did not develop satiety but continued to eat for hours. The sham feeding paradigm has demonstrated the important role of orosensory stimuli in ingestion. Increasing the concentration of sugar solutions or oil emulsions increases the amount consumed in a linear fashion over extensive concentration ranges.[65–67] Sham feeding does eventually stop and a number of processes have been proposed to contribute to the cessation of sham feeding including oral metering,[68] habituation[69] and sensory-specific satiety (decreasing the pleasantness of a specific food as more is ingested).[70]

In normal ingestion, consumed nutrients contact gastrointestinal mechanosensitive and chemosensitive receptors that provide feedback information that is important to the control of meal size. The potential range of feedback mechanisms that could be operating to lead to meal termination depends on the distribution of ingested nutrients during the meal. During eating, gastric emptying is more rapid than after a meal,[71,72] meaning that before meal termination, ingested nutrients not only accumulate within the stomach but also come into contact with a significant portion of the small intestine. Thus, the stomach and the upper small intestine are potential sites for the generation of signals providing feedback on the nature and quantity of consumed nutrients.

The vagus nerve (cranial nerve X) is the major neuroanatomic link between the gastrointestinal tract and brain.[73] Vagal afferent fibers with cell bodies in the nodose ganglion innervate the digestive organs and project to the NTS in the dorsal hindbrain with a rough viscerotopic representation of the alimentary canal.[74] The response properties of vagal afferent fibers depend in part on the target organ they innervate. Mechanosensitive gastric vagal afferents increase their firing in response to increasing gastric load volume.[75] Individual afferent fibers are differentially tuned such that there are differences in their dynamic range.[76] Some afferents reach their maximal activity at small intragastric volumes, whereas others do not begin to respond until a significant gastric load is present. Gastric mechanoreceptive vagal afferent fibers do not respond directly to the nutrient character of the gastric contents. Firing rates are similarly increased by nutrient and nonnutrient load volumes.[77] In contrast, duodenal vagal afferents are activated by both the volume and nutrient character of intestinal contents.[78,79] Although gastric vagal activity is not responsive directly to intragastric nutrient character, gastric afferent responsivity can be altered by the presence of duodenal nutrients.[80]

Alterations in vagal afferent activity may be stimulated by nutrient induced release of a range of gastrointestinal peptides. For example, the brain/gut peptide cholecystokinin (CCK) is released by the duodenal presence of nutrient digestion products. Duodenal vagal afferents that express CCK receptors[81] are activated by local CCK administration and combinations of duodenal load and CCK combine to produce greater duodenal vagal afferent activity than either alone.[82] CCK also plays a role in the response of duodenal vagal afferents to duodenal nutrients.[78] CCK administration results in increases in vagal gastric mechanoreceptive afferent activity similar to those produced by intragastric load[83] and, again, combinations of gastric load and CCK produce greater degrees of activity than either alone.[83] Experiments with CCK receptor antagonists have demonstrated that endogenous CCK plays a role in the response of duodenal afferents to nutrients.[78]

Elimination of aspects of vagal afferent or peptide-induced feedback can result in significant alterations in meal patterns. For example, surgical vagal deafferentation results in the consumption of larger meals than those consumed by sham operated controls.[84] The number of meals consumed during the day is reduced in response to these meal size increases such that overall food intake is unchanged. Similar alterations in meal size also occur in response to the administration of CCK antagonists.[85,86]

A number of peripherally acting peptides with roles in the control of eating have been identified. The best characterized of these is the brain–gut peptide CCK. CCK is released from I cells in the upper intestine in response to the presence of intraluminal nutrients. Exogenously administered CCK was originally demonstrated to decrease food intake in rats[87] and this feeding inhibitory action of CCK and CCK agonists has been demonstrated in a range of species including nonhuman primates and man.[88,89] Exogenously administered CCK reduces meal size and results in an earlier appearance of a behavioral satiety sequence.[90] A role for CCK in the control of the size of individual meals was confirmed by experiments examining the effects of repeated, meal-contingent administration of CCK. CCK consistently reduces meal size without producing a significant change in overall daily food intake.[91]

As discussed, CCK activates vagal afferents. Disruption of subdiaphragmatic vagal afferent signaling significantly blunts the ability of CCK to inhibit food intake.[92-94] A role for endogenous CCK in satiety is supported by data demonstrating that administration of CCK antagonists with specificity for the CCK-1 receptor result in increased food intake. This increase is almost completely accounted for by an increase in the size of their first meal.[86] Alterations in meal patterns are also evident in rats lacking CCK-1 receptors—Otsuka Long Evans Tokushima Fatty (OLETF) rats.[95] OLETF rats are obese and hyperphagic. Characterization of their spontaneous solid or liquid food intake has revealed overall increases in daily food intake that are expressed through significant increases in the size of individual meals with an incomplete compensation in meal number.[96]

Satiety actions for the pancreatic peptides glucagon and amylin have also been demonstrated. Eating rapidly elicits an increase in pancreatic glucagon secretion.[97] Glucagon is cleared rapidly from the circulation by the liver[97] and the liver seems to be the site of glucagon's satiety action.[98] Hepatic–portal infusion of glucagon at meal onset elicits a dose-related reduction in meal size[99] and the satiety action requires the presence of other forms of ingestional consequences because glucagon does not affect intake during sham feeding.[100] The satiety action of pancreatic glucagon is mediated vagally; transection of the hepatic branch of the vagus blocks glucagon satiety.[101] A role for endogenous glucagon in the control of meal size is supported by data demonstrating the ability of hepatic portal infusions of glucagon antibody to increase meal size.[102]

Amylin is cosecreted with insulin from pancreatic beta cells. Amylin plasma levels increase rapidly with meal onset and remain increased for a significant period of time during and after meals. Exogenously administered amylin inhibits feeding in a dose-dependent and behaviorally specific manner.[103] Amylin's primary site of action is within the area postrema, a hindbrain structure lacking a blood–brain barrier,[104] although recent work has suggested actions in multiple brain areas to affect food intake.[105] A physiologic role for endogenous amylin in feeding controls is supported by experiments demonstrating increases in food intake in response to administration of amylin antagonists.[106]

Both peptide YY (3-36) [PYY(3-36)] and glucagon-like peptide 1 (GLP-1) are secreted from intestinal L cells in response to the intraluminal presence of nutrients. In contrast with CCK, the secretion of PYY and GLP-1 is maintained after meal termination, suggesting roles for these peptides in feeding control beyond the individual meal. Exogenously administered PYY 3-36 has been shown to inhibit food intake in multiple species including man.[107-109] The feeding inhibitory actions of PYY are likely mediated through interactions with the inhibitory Y2 receptors on NPY/AgRP neurons.[107,110] Further supporting a brain site of action, PYY 3-36 administration has been shown to modulate patterns of cortical and hypothalamic neuronal activation in human subjects consistent with its actions in inhibiting food intake.[111] Exogenously administered GLP-1 or long-acting GLP-1 receptor agonists inhibit food intake. Meal-contingent GLP-1 administration leads to earlier meal termination and thus reductions in meal size.[112] Prolonged GLP-1 infusions or administration of long acting GLP-1 analogs reduce overall food intake and do so through reductions in meal size.[113,114] Examinations of a role for endogenous GLP-1 in the controls of meal size have produced mixed results[115,116] questioning whether meal stimulated intestinal GLP-1 release is involved in meal termination under normal circmstances. Circulating GLP-1 is degraded rapidly by dipeptidyl peptidase-IV (DPP-IV) making it unlikely that feeding actions of the normally released peptide are mediated through endocrine mechanisms.[117] GLP-1 receptors are expressed in vagal afferent neurons and total subdiaphragmatic or specific afferent vagotomy has been demonstrated to significantly attenuate the satiety effects of intraperitoneally administered GLP-1. Thus, meal released GLP-1 may act on vagal afferent terminals in close approximation to the enteroendocrine L cells to affect food intake.

As well as deriving from the lower intestine, GLP-1 is also expressed in neurons within the NTS.[118] These neurons project extensively throughout the brain including to a variety of hypothalamic and reward sites.[119] Centrally administered GLP-1 inhibits food intake, although the effects are site specific.[120] For example, GLP-1 administered into the amygdala not only reduces food intake, but also induces a conditioned taste aversion, whereas GLP-1 administration to hypothalamic, hindbrain, or reward sites seems to have specific feeding inhibitory actions.[120–123] Whether gut-released GLP-1 affects feeding through activation of specific brain targets has not been investigated adequately. However, GLP-1 and GLP-1 analogs have been demonstrated to readily cross the blood–brain barrier[124] and, thus, degradation-resistant GLP-1 analogs or the high circulating levels found after bariatric surgery likely access central sites to inhibit food intake.[125]

Unlike these peptides that limit food intake, ghrelin, a brain–gut peptide that is primarily synthesized in the stomach, stimulates food intake after either peripheral or central administration.[126,127] Ghrelin synthesis and plasma ghrelin levels are increased by food deprivation and reduced by refeeding,[126] and this pattern of release in relation to meals is consistent with a role for ghrelin in meal initiation.[128] Repeated exogenous ghrelin administration can result in obesity[129] and ghrelin antagonists have been shown to reduce food intake, supporting a role for the endogenous peptide in stimulating eating.[130] Arcuate NPY/AgRP–containing neurons express ghrelin receptors[131] and peripheral or central ghrelin administration increases arcuate NPY expression,[132–134] suggesting a hypothalamic site of action. However, ghrelin has also been shown to increase food intake when administered in the hindbrain, leading to the suggestion that ghrelin's actions are distributed across multiple brain sites.[132,135] Knockout of either ghrelin or its receptor protects against a high-fat diet–induced obesity[136,137] and the double knockout results in mice with a lean phenotype.[138]

As well as being modulated by short-term feeding status, plasma ghrelin levels are affected by long-term energy status or adiposity. Thus, ghrelin levels are lower in obesity and increase in response to weight loss.[139] Together with the short-term effects of ghrelin on arcuate NPY, these data suggest a role for ghrelin that opposes that of leptin on overall arcuate signaling.

REWARD SIGNALING

As noted, food choice and the amounts consumed are greatly affected by taste or palatability. The effects of palatability on ingestion have been shown to have both opioid and dopaminergic mediation. Opiate agonists increase, whereas antagonists decrease, eating and these effects on ingestion seem to occur through alterations in palatability. Morphine enhances the intake of preferred over nonpreferred diets[140] and enhances hedonic responses to sweet solutions.[141] In contrast, administration of the opioid antagonist naloxone specifically reduces the intake of a preferred diet while not affecting the intake of a nonpreferred diet in a choice paradigm.[142]

A major site of action for opioids in modulating palatability is the nucleus accumbens (NAc). Microinjections of opioid agonists into the medial shell region of the NAc increase both ingestion and positive responses in taste reactivity tests.[143–145] Furthermore, in a paradigm in which recently consumed tastes are less preferred, NAc injections of opioid agonists increase and antagonists decrease the consumption of a prefed flavor, again suggesting modulation of palatability.[146]

Dopaminergic mediation of palatability has also been documented. Dopamine agonists increase eating[147] and animals with severe neurotoxin-induced dopamine depletions[148] or dopamine deficient through gene knockout[149] fail to consume food independently. Feeding increases extracellular dopamine within the NAc[150] and the increase is greater with the consumption of a highly palatable food,[151] suggesting a role for mesolimbic dopamine in mediating food reward. Such increases can also be shown in response to sham feeding of sucrose or corn oil demonstrating that taste is a sufficient stimulus for increased NAc dopamine release,[152,153] suggesting that dopamine plays a critical role in the hedonic processing of orosensory stimuli.

Not only the taste but also the nutrient consequences of ingestion can serve to reinforce dietary choice. This is best demonstrated in experiments that pair a novel noncaloric taste with an intragastric nutrient infusion. Animals come to prefer a taste that has been associated with an intragastric nutrient. Although the phenomenon of flavor conditioning is well-documented, its mediation is not well-understood. Feedback pathways that mediate satiety do not seem to be involved.[154] In contrast with the mediation of palatability, nutrient conditioning does not seem to depend on opioid mediation.[155] However, dopaminergic mediation is required because D1 receptor antagonists block or significantly attenuate the acquisition of preferences to a flavor paired with gastric nutrients[156,157] and this seems to involve a separate population of dopaminergic neurons from those that encode palatability.[158]

INTERACTIONS AMONG SIGNALING SYSTEMS

Although the controls of eating depend on these seemingly separate systems, an important issue is where and how these systems interact to control meals and overall intake. A number of the clearest demonstrations of interactions involve the adiposity signal leptin. Both peripheral and central leptin administration reduce food intake and leptin's effects on eating are expressed as reductions in meal size without changing meal frequency.[159–161] Leptin's actions in reducing meal size depend in part on interactions with satiety signals. For example, administration of leptin at doses that are subthreshold for inhibiting eating when administered alone, enhance the satiating potential of peripheral CCK or an intragastric nutrient preload.[162–164] This action of leptin seems to depend on its ability to enhance the NTS neural activation produced feedback satiety signaling. That is, leptin enhances the dorsal hindbrain representation of ascending vagal afferent feedback signals arising from CCK or gastric preload induced gastrointestinal stimulation.[165] Reducing leptin levels through food deprivation or exogenous NPY administration have the opposite result - the satiating potency of CCK is reduced[166,167] and satiety related NTS activation is inhibited.[165] These actions of leptin may be a downstream consequence of leptin signaling in the arcuate nucleus or directly mediated at hindbrain sites since the NTS contains receptors for both leptin and NPY.[168,169]

Leptin may also decrease meal size by altering the reinforcing effects of ingestion. Leptin receptors are located on ventral tegmental area (VTA) dopamine neurons[170] as well as on lateral hypothalamic neurotensin neurons that project to the VTA and leptin can regulate the activity of VTA.[171] The outcome of such interactions impacts overall reward signaling. Thus, leptin reduces the rewarding efficacy of electrical brain self stimulation[172] and reduces conditioned place preferences to rewarding foods.[173] In contrast, ghrelin has been demonstrated to enhance the rewarding value of high fat diets as reflected in conditioned preferences.[174] Similar effects on reward pathways have been demonstrated for insulin.[175] Thus, adiposity signals serving as long term regulators of energy balance have multiple actions. Many of these may contribute to the controls food intake in ways that both modulate the negative feedback effects of ingestion while also affecting positive feedback. Together these actions result in the modulation of meal size that, over the long term, contribute to the maintenance of energy balance.

Satiety signals can also affect the efficacy of adiposity signals. For example, CCK has been demonstrated to enhance the ability of leptin to reduce food intake and decrease body weight over the longer term.[176–178] In addition, the satiety signal amylin alters leptin sensitivity, restoring responsivity to exogenous leptin in diet induced obese animals that are otherwise leptin resistant.[179,180] Satiety signals can also affect reward processing. As noted above, GLP-1 receptors are found in both the VTA and the NAc and administration of GLP-1 or GLP-1 agonists to these brain areas reduces food intake and does so in ways consistent with reduced reward.[122,181] Similarly, amylin receptor subunits are expressed in the VTA and amylin administration at this site reduces intake and does so by modulating VTA dopaminergic signaling.[182] Amylin receptors are also expressed in the shell region of the NAc and amylin administration can reverse μ-opioid induced feeding through actions at this site.[183]

Finally, alterations in reward signaling can modulate hypothalamic systems involved in feeding control. Palatable diet intake stimulated by NAc μ-opioid agonist administration depends upon activation of multiple hypothalamic sites and suppression of activity in these sites blocks this feeding.[184] Roles for both orexin and NPY in mediating the effects of NAc μ-opioid induced feeding have been demonstrated.[185,186]

SUMMARY

There are multiple physiologic and neural systems involved in controlling eating. These systems derive from and control different aspects of ingestive behavior and its consequences. While adiposity, satiety and reward signaling have different primary sites of mediation within the brain, these are interacting systems that together modulate food intake. Some of the currently approved pharmacotherapies aimed at reducing eating and body weight target these signaling systems. For example, liraglutide, the active ingredient in Saxenda is a GLP-1 agonist compound targeting satiety signaling, Contrave contains the opioid antagonist naltrexone, targeting reward signaling and locaserin in Belviq is a serotonin agonist thought to act on POMC neurons that contribute to adiposity responses.

REFERENCES

1. Coleman DL. Effect of parabiosis of obese and diabetes and normal mice. Diabetologia 1973;9:194–298.

2. Zhang Y, Proenca R, Maffei M, et al. Positional cloning of the mouse obese gene and its human homologue. Nature 1994;372(6505):425–32.

3. Tartaglia LA, Dembski M, Weng X, et al. Identification and expression cloning of a leptin receptor, OB-R. Cell 1995;83(7):1263–71.

4. Chua SC Jr, Chung WK, Wu-Peng XS, et al. Phenotypes of mouse diabetes and rat fatty due to mutations in the OB (leptin) receptor. Science 1996;271(5251): 994–6.

5. Maffei M, Halaas J, Ravussin E, et al. Leptin levels in human and rodent: measurement of plasma leptin and ob RNA in obese and weight-reduced subjects. Nat Med 1995;1(11):1155–61.

6. Elmquist JK, Bjørbaek C, Ahima RS, et al. Distributions of leptin receptor mRNA isoforms in the rat brain. J Comp Neurol 1998;395(4):535–47.

7. Schwartz MW, Seeley RJ, Campfield LA, et al. Identification of targets of leptin action in rat hypothalamus. J Clin Invest 1996;98(5):1101–6.

8. Elias CF, Aschkenasi C, Lee C, et al. Leptin differentially regulates NPY and POMC neurons projecting to the lateral hypothalamic area. Neuron 1999; 23(4):775–86.

9. Fan W, Boston BA, Kesterson RA, et al. Role of melanocortinergic neurons in feeding and the agouti obesity syndrome. Nature 1997;385(6612):165–8.

10. Thiele TE, van Dijk G, Yagaloff KA, et al. Central infusion of melanocortin agonist MTII in rats: assessment of c-Fos expression and taste aversion. Am J Physiol 1998;274(1 Pt 2):R248–54.

11. Cowley MA, Smart JL, Rubinstein M, et al. Leptin activates anorexigenic POMC neurons through a neural network in the arcuate nucleus. Nature 2001; 411(6836):480–4.

12. Schwartz MW, Seeley RJ, Woods SC, et al. Leptin increases hypothalamic pro-opiomelanocortin mRNA expression in the rostral arcuate nucleus. Diabetes 1997;46(12):2119–23.

13. Enriori PJ, Evans AE, Sinnayah P, et al. Diet-induced obesity causes severe but reversible leptin resistance in arcuate melanocortin neurons. Cell Metab 2007; 5(3):181–94.

14. Kim EM, Welch CC, Grace MK, et al. Chronic food restriction and acute food deprivation decrease mRNA levels of opioid peptides in arcuate nucleus. Am J Physiol 1996;270(5 Pt 2):R1019–24.

15. Hagan MM, Rushing PA, Schwartz MW, et al. Role of the CNS melanocortin system in the response to overfeeding. J Neurosci 1999;19(6):2362–7.

16. Challis BG, Coll AP, Yeo GS, et al. Mice lacking pro-opiomelanocortin are sensitive to high-fat feeding but respond normally to the acute anorectic effects of peptide-YY(3-36). Proc Natl Acad Sci U S A 2004;101(13):4695–700.

17. Butler AA, Cone RD. The melanocortin receptors: lessons from knockout models. Neuropeptides 2002;36(2–3):77–84.

18. Farooqi IS, O'Rahilly S. Mutations in ligands and receptors of the leptin-melanocortin pathway that lead to obesity. Nat Clin Pract Endocrinol Metab 2008;4(10):569–77.

19. Luquet S, Perez FA, Hnasko TS, et al. NPY/AgRP neurons are essential for feeding in adult mice but can be ablated in neonates. Science 2005; 310(5748):683–5.

20. Levine AS, Morley JE. Neuropeptide Y: a potent inducer of consummatory behavior in rats. Peptides 1984;5(6):1025–9.

21. Clark J, Kalra PS, Crowley WR, et al. Neuropeptide Y and human pancreatic polypeptide stimulate feeding behavior in rats. Endocrinology 1984;115(1): 427–9.

22. Stanley BG, Magdalin W, Seirafi A, et al. The perifornical area: the major focus of (a) patchily distributed hypothalamic neuropeptide Y-sensitive feeding system(s). Brain Res 1993;604(1–2):304–17.

23. Stanley BG, Daniel DR, Chin AS, et al. Paraventricular nucleus injections of pep-tide YY and neuropeptide Y preferentially enhance carbohydrate ingestion. Pep-tides 1985;6(6):1205–11.

24. Gehlert DR, Chronwall BM, Schafer MP, et al. Localization of neuropeptide Y messenger ribonucleic acid in rat and mouse brain by in situ hybridization. Syn-apse 1987;1(1):25–31.

25. Tiesjema B, la Fleur SE, Luijendijk MC, et al. Sustained NPY overexpression in the PVN results in obesity via temporarily increasing food intake. Obesity (Silver Spring) 2009;17(7):1448–50.

26. Yang L, Scott KA, Hyun J, et al. Role of dorsomedial hypothalamic neuropeptide Y in modulating food intake and energy balance. J Neurosci 2009;29(1):179–90.

27. Hahn TM, Breininger JF, Baskin DG, et al. Coexpression of Agrp and NPY in fasting-activated hypothalamic neurons. Nat Neurosci 1998;1(4):271–2.

28. Grill HJ, Ginsberg AB, Seeley RJ, et al. Brainstem application of melanocortin receptor ligands produces long-lasting effects on feeding and body weight. J Neurosci 1998;18(23):10128–35.

29. Wu Q, Boyle MP, Palmiter RD. Loss of GABAergic signaling by AgRP neurons to the parabrachial nucleus leads to starvation. Cell 2009;137(7):1225–34.

30. van Dijk G, Seeley RJ, Thiele TE, et al. Metabolic, gastrointestinal, and CNS neu-ropeptide effects of brain leptin administration in the rat. Am J Physiol 1999; 276(5 Pt 2):R1425–33.

31. Masaki T, Yoshimichi G, Chiba S, et al. Corticotropin-releasing hormone-mediated pathway of leptin to regulate feeding, adiposity, and uncoupling pro-tein expression in mice. Endocrinology 2003;144(8):3547–54.

32. Lu XY, Barsh GS, Akil H, et al. Interaction between alpha-melanocyte-stimulating hormone and corticotropin-releasing hormone in the regulation of feeding and hypothalamo-pituitary-adrenal responses. J Neurosci 2003;23(21):7863–72.

33. Blevins JE, Schwartz MW, Baskin DG. Evidence that paraventricular nucleus oxytocin neurons link hypothalamic leptin action to caudal brainstem nuclei con-trolling meal size. Am J Physiol Regul Integr Comp Physiol 2004;287(1):R87–96.

34. Ladenheim EE, Behles RR, Bi S, et al. Gastrin-releasing peptide messenger ri-bonucleic acid expression in the hypothalamic paraventricular nucleus is altered by melanocortin receptor stimulation and food deprivation. Endocri-nology 2009;150(2):672–8.

35. Levine AS, Rogers B, Kneip J, et al. Effect of centrally administered corticotropin releasing factor (CRF) on multiple feeding paradigms. Neuropharmacology 1983;22(3):337–9.

36. Ladenheim EE, Taylor JE, Coy DH, et al. Hindbrain GRP receptor blockade an-tagonizes feeding suppression by peripherally administered GRP. Am J Physiol 1996;271(1 Pt 2):R180–4.

37. Arletti R, Benelli A, Bertolini A. Influence of oxytocin on feeding behavior in the rat. Peptides 1989;10(1):89–93.

38. Lopez M, Seoane L, García MC, et al. Leptin regulation of prepro-orexin and orexin receptor mRNA levels in the hypothalamus. Biochem Biophys Res Com-mun 2000;269(1):41–5.

39. Perez-Leighton CE, Boland K, Teske JA, et al. Behavioral responses to orexin, orexin receptor gene expression, and spontaneous physical activity contribute to individual sensitivity to obesity. Am J Physiol Endocrinol Metab 2012; 303(7):E865–74.

40. Haynes AC, Jackson B, Chapman H, et al. A selective orexin-1 receptor antagonist reduces food consumption in male and female rats. Regul Pept 2000; 96(1–2):45–51.

41. Qu D, Ludwig DS, Gammeltoft S, et al. A role for melanin-concentrating hormone in the central regulation of feeding behaviour. Nature 1996;380(6571): 243–7.

42. Sahu A. Evidence suggesting that galanin (GAL), melanin-concentrating hormone (MCH), neurotensin (NT), proopiomelanocortin (POMC) and neuropeptide Y (NPY) are targets of leptin signaling in the hypothalamus. Endocrinology 1998; 139(2):795–8.

43. Rossi M, Choi SJ, O'Shea D, et al. Melanin-concentrating hormone acutely stimulates feeding, but chronic administration has no effect on body weight. Endocrinology 1997;138(1):351–5.

44. Ludwig DS, Tritos NA, Mastaitis JW, et al. Melanin-concentrating hormone overexpression in transgenic mice leads to obesity and insulin resistance. J Clin Invest 2001;107(3):379–86.

45. Corp ES, Woods SC, Porte D Jr, et al. Localization of 125I-insulin binding sites in the rat hypothalamus by quantitative autoradiography. Neurosci Lett 1986;70(1): 17–22.

46. Woods SC, Lotter EC, McKay LD, et al. Chronic intracerebroventricular infusion of insulin reduces food intake and body weight of baboons. Nature 1979; 282(5738):503–5.

47. Schwartz MW, Sipols AJ, Marks JL, et al. Inhibition of hypothalamic neuropeptide Y gene expression by insulin. Endocrinology 1992;130(6):3608–16.

48. Xu AW, Kaelin CB, Takeda K, et al. PI3K integrates the action of insulin and leptin on hypothalamic neurons. J Clin Invest 2005;115(4):951–8.

49. Moran TH. Hypothalamic nutrient sensing and energy balance. Forum Nutr 2010;63:94–101.

50. Levin BE, Dunn-Meynell AA, Routh VH. Brain glucosensing and the K(ATP) channel. Nat Neurosci 2001;4(5):459–60.

51. Levin B. Neuronal glucose sensing: still a physiological orphan. Cell Metab 2007;6:252–4.

52. Dunn-Meynell AA, Sanders NM, Compton D, et al. Relationship among brain and blood glucose levels and spontaneous and glucoprivic feeding. J Neurosci 2009;29(21):7015–22.

53. Le Foll C, Irani BG, Magnan C, et al. Characteristics and mechanisms of hypothalamic neuronal fatty acid sensing. Am J Physiol Regul Integr Comp Physiol 2009;297(3):R655–64.

54. Oomura Y, Nakamura T, Sugimori M, et al. Effect of free fatty acid on the rat lateral hypothalamic neurons. Physiol Behav 1975;14(04):483–6.

55. Obici S, Feng Z, Morgan K, et al. Central administration of oleic acid inhibits glucose production and food intake. Diabetes 2002;51(2):271–5.

56. Obici S, Rossetti L. Minireview: nutrient sensing and the regulation of insulin action and energy balance. Endocrinology 2003;144(12):5172–8.

57. Cota D, Proulx K, Smith KA, et al. Hypothalamic mTOR signaling regulates food intake. Science 2006;312(5775):927–30.

58. Morrison CD, Xi X, White CL, et al. Amino acids inhibit Agrp gene expression via an mTOR-dependent mechanism. Am J Physiol Endocrinol Metab 2007;293(1): E165–71.

59. Huo L, Maeng L, Bjørbaek C, et al. Leptin and the control of food intake: neurons in the nucleus of the solitary tract are activated by both gastric distension and leptin. Endocrinology 2007;148(5):2189–97.

60. Hayes MR, Skibicka KP, Bence KK, et al. Dorsal hindbrain 5′-adenosine monophosphate-activated protein kinase as an intracellular mediator of energy balance. Endocrinology 2009;150(5):2175–82.

61. Hayes MR, Skibicka KP, Leichner TM, et al. Endogenous leptin signaling in the caudal nucleus tractus solitarius and area postrema is required for energy balance regulation. Cell Metab 2010;11(1):77–83.

62. Grill HJ, Hayes MR. The nucleus tractus solitarius: a portal for visceral afferent signal processing, energy status assessment and integration of their combined effects on food intake. Int J Obes (Lond) 2009;33(Suppl 1):S11–5.

63. Grill HJ. Distributed neural control of energy balance: contributions from hindbrain and hypothalamus. Obesity (Silver Spring) 2006;14(Suppl 5):216S–21S.

64. Pavlov I. The work of the digestiver glands. London: Charles Griffin and Co, Ltd; 1910.

65. Mook D. Oral and postingestional determinants of various solutions in rats with esophageal fistulas. J Comp Physiol Psychol 1963;56:645–59.

66. Weingarten HP, Watson SD. Sham feeding as a procedure for assessing the influence of diet palatability on food intake. Physiol Behav 1982;28(3):401–7.

67. Grill HJ, Kaplan JM. Sham feeding in intact and chronic decerebrate rats. Am J Physiol 1992;262(6 Pt 2):R1070–4.

68. Mook D. Satiety, specifications and stop rules: feeding as a voluntary act. In: Epstein A, Morrison AR, editors. Progress in psychobiology and physiological psychology. New York: Academic Press; 1990. p. 1–65.

69. Swithers SE, Hall WG. Does oral experience terminate ingestion? Appetite 1994; 23(2):113–38.

70. Rolls BJ. Sensory-specific satiety. Nutr Rev 1986;44(3):93–101.

71. Kaplan JM, Spector AC, Grill HJ. Dynamics of gastric emptying during and after stomach fill. Am J Physiol 1992;263(4 Pt 2):R813–9.

72. Moran TH, Knipp S, Schwartz GJ. Gastric and duodenal features of meals mediate controls of liquid gastric emptying during fill in rhesus monkeys. Am J Physiol 1999;277(5 Pt 2):R1282–90.

73. Prechtl JC, Powley TL. Organization and distribution of the rat subdiaphragmatic vagus and associated paraganglia. J Comp Neurol 1985;235(2):182–95.

74. Altschuler SM, Bao XM, Bieger D, et al. Viscerotopic representation of the upper alimentary tract in the rat: sensory ganglia and nuclei of the solitary and spinal trigeminal tracts. J Comp Neurol 1989;283(2):248–68.

75. Andrews PL, Grundy D, Scratcherd T. Vagal afferent discharge from mechanoreceptors in different regions of the ferret stomach. J Physiol 1980;298:513–24.

76. Schwartz GJ, McHugh PR, Moran TH. Gastric loads and cholecystokinin synergistically stimulate rat gastric vagal afferents. Am J Physiol 1993;265(4 Pt 2): R872–6.

77. Mathis C, Moran TH, Schwartz GJ. Load-sensitive rat gastric vagal afferents encode volume but not gastric nutrients. Am J Physiol 1998;274(2 Pt 2):R280–6.

78. Eastwood C, Maubach K, Kirkup AJ, et al. The role of endogenous cholecystokinin in the sensory transduction of luminal nutrient signals in the rat jejunum. Neurosci Lett 1998;254(3):145–8.

79. Randich A, Tyler WJ, Cox JE, et al. Responses of celiac and cervical vagal afferents to infusions of lipids in the jejunum or ileum of the rat. Am J Physiol Regul Integr Comp Physiol 2000;278(1):R34–43.

80. Schwartz GJ, Moran TH. Duodenal nutrient exposure elicits nutrient-specific gut motility and vagal afferent signals in rat. Am J Physiol 1998;274(5 Pt 2): R1236–42.

81. Moran TH, Norgren R, Crosby RJ, et al. Central and peripheral vagal transport of cholecystokinin binding sites occurs in afferent fibers. Brain Res 1990;526(1): 95–102.

82. Schwartz GJ, Tougas G, Moran TH. Integration of vagal afferent responses to duodenal loads and exogenous CCK in rats. Peptides 1995;16(4):707–11.

83. Schwartz GJ, McHugh PR, Moran TH. Integration of vagal afferent responses to gastric loads and cholecystokinin in rats. Am J Physiol 1991;261(1 Pt 2):R64–9.

84. Schwartz GJ, Salorio CF, Skoglund C, et al. Gut vagal afferent lesions increase meal size but do not block gastric preload-induced feeding suppression. Am J Physiol 1999;276(6 Pt 2):R1623–9.

85. Moran TH, Ameglio PJ, Schwartz GJ, et al. Blockade of type A, not type B, CCK receptors attenuates satiety actions of exogenous and endogenous CCK. Am J Physiol 1992;262(1 Pt 2):R46–50.

86. Moran TH, Ameglio PJ, Peyton HJ, et al. Blockade of type A, but not type B, CCK receptors postpones satiety in rhesus monkeys. Am J Physiol 1993; 265(3 Pt 2):R620–4.

87. Gibbs J, Young RC, Smith GP. Cholecystokinin decreases food intake in rats. J Comp Physiol Psychol 1973;84(3):488–95.

88. Pi-Sunyer X, Kissileff HR, Thornton J, et al. C-terminal octapeptide of cholecystokinin decreases food intake in obese men. Physiol Behav 1982;29(4):627–30.

89. Moran TH, McHugh PR. Cholecystokinin suppresses food intake by inhibiting gastric emptying. Am J Physiol 1982;242(5):R491–7.

90. Antin J, Giibs J, Jolt J, et al. Cholecystokinin elicits the complete behavioral sequence of satiety in rats. J Comp Physiol Psychol 1975;89:784–90.

91. West DB, Fey D, Woods SC. Cholecystokinin persistently suppresses meal size but not food intake in free-feeding rats. Am J Physiol 1984;246(5 Pt 2):R776–87.

92. Smith G, Jerome C, Norgren R. Afferent axons in the abdominal vagus mediate the satiety effects of cholecystokinin in rats. Am J Physiol 1985;249:R638–41.

93. Ritter RC, Ladenheim EE. Capsaicin pretreatment attenuates suppression of food intake by cholecystokinin. Am J Physiol 1985;248(4 Pt 2):R501–4.

94. Moran TH, Baldessarini AR, Salorio CF, et al. Vagal afferent and efferent contributions to the inhibition of food intake by cholecystokinin. Am J Physiol 1997; 272(4 Pt 2):R1245–51.

95. Takiguchi S, Takata Y, Funakoshi A, et al. Disrupted cholecystokinin type-A receptor (CCKAR) gene in OLETF rats. Gene 1997;197(1–2):169–75.

96. Moran TH, Katz LF, Plata-Salaman CR, et al. Disordered food intake and obesity in rats lacking cholecystokinin A receptors. Am J Physiol 1998;274(3 Pt 2): R618–25.

97. Langhans W, Pantel K, Müller-Schell W, et al. Hepatic handling of pancreatic glucagon and glucose during meals in rats. Am J Physiol 1984;247(5 Pt 2): R827–32.

98. Geary N. Glucagon and the control of meal size. In: Smith G, editor. Satiation: from gut to brain. New York: Oxford University Press; 1998. p. 164–97.

99. Geary N, Le Sauter J, Noh U. Glucagon acts in the liver to control spontaneous meal size in rats. Am J Physiol 1993;264(1 Pt 2):R116–22.

100. Geary N, Smith GP. Pancreatic glucagon fails to inhibit sham feeding in the rat. Peptides 1982;3(2):163–6.

101. Geary N, Smith GP. Selective hepatic vagotomy blocks pancreatic glucagon's satiety effect. Physiol Behav 1983;31(3):391–4.
102. Le Sauter J, Noh U, Geary N. Hepatic portal infusion of glucagon antibodies increases spontaneous meal size in rats. Am J Physiol 1991;261(1 Pt 2):R162–5.
103. Lutz TA, Geary N, Szabady MM, et al. Amylin decreases meal size in rats. Physiol Behav 1995;58(6):1197–202.
104. Lutz TA, Senn M, Althaus J, et al. Lesion of the area postrema/nucleus of the solitary tract (AP/NTS) attenuates the anorectic effects of amylin and calcitonin gene-related peptide (CGRP) in rats. Peptides 1998;19(2):309–17.
105. Mietlicki-Baase EG, Hayes MR. Amylin activates distributed CNS nuclei to control energy balance. Physiol Behav 2014;136:39–46.
106. Rushing PA, Hagan MM, Seeley RJ, et al. Inhibition of central amylin signaling increases food intake and body adiposity in rats. Endocrinology 2001; 142(11):5035.
107. Batterham RL, Cowley MA, Small CJ, et al. Gut hormone PYY(3-36) physiologically inhibits food intake. Nature 2002;418(6898):650–4.
108. Batterham RL, Cohen MA, Ellis SM, et al. Inhibition of food intake in obese subjects by peptide YY3-36. N Engl J Med 2003;349(10):941–8.
109. Moran TH, Smedh U, Kinzig KP, et al. Peptide YY (3-36) inhibits gastric emptying and produces acute reductions in food intake in rhesus monkeys. Am J Physiol Regul Integr Comp Physiol 2005;288(2):R384–8.
110. Keire DA, Mannon P, Kobayashi M, et al. Primary structures of PYY, [Pro(34)] PYY, and PYY-(3-36) confer different conformations and receptor selectivity. Am J Physiol Gastrointest Liver Physiol 2000;279(1):G126–31.
111. Batterham RL, ffytche DH, Rosenthal JM, et al. PYY modulation of cortical and hypothalamic brain areas predicts feeding behaviour in humans. Nature 2007; 450(7166):106–9.
112. Ruttimann EB, Arnold M, Hillebrand JJ, et al. Intrameal hepatic portal and intraperitoneal infusions of glucagon-like peptide-1 reduce spontaneous meal size in the rat via different mechanisms. Endocrinology 2009;150(3):1174–81.
113. Chelikani PK, Haver AC, Reidelberger RD. Intravenous infusion of glucagon-like peptide-1 potently inhibits food intake, sham feeding, and gastric emptying in rats. Am J Physiol Regul Integr Comp Physiol 2005;288(6):R1695–706.
114. Scott KA, Moran TH. The GLP-1 agonist exendin-4 reduces food intake in non-human primates through changes in meal size. Am J Physiol Regul Integr Comp Physiol 2007;293(3):R983–7.
115. Ruttimann EB, Arnold M, Geary N, et al. GLP-1 antagonism with exendin (9-39) fails to increase spontaneous meal size in rats. Physiol Behav 2010;100(4): 291–6.
116. Williams DL, Baskin DG, Schwartz MW. Evidence that intestinal glucagon-like peptide-1 plays a physiological role in satiety. Endocrinology 2009;150(4): 1680–7.
117. Kieffer TJ, McIntosh CH, Pederson RA. Degradation of glucose-dependent insulinotropic polypeptide and truncated glucagon-like peptide 1 in vitro and in vivo by dipeptidyl peptidase IV. Endocrinology 1995;136(8):3585–96.
118. Han VK, Hynes MA, Jin C, et al. Cellular localization of proglucagon/glucagon-like peptide I messenger RNAs in rat brain. J Neurosci Res 1986;16(1):97–107.
119. Goke R, Larsen PJ, Mikkelsen JD, et al. Distribution of GLP-1 binding sites in the rat brain: evidence that exendin-4 is a ligand of brain GLP-1 binding sites. Eur J Neurosci 1995;7(11):2294–300.

120. Kinzig KP, D'Alessio DA, Seeley RJ. The diverse roles of specific GLP-1 receptors in the control of food intake and the response to visceral illness. J Neurosci 2002;22(23):10470–6.

121. Kinzig KP, D'Alessio DA, Herman JP, et al. CNS glucagon-like peptide-1 receptors mediate endocrine and anxiety responses to interoceptive and psychogenic stressors. J Neurosci 2003;23(15):6163–70.

122. Dossat AM, Diaz R, Gallo L, et al. Nucleus accumbens GLP-1 receptors influence meal size and palatability. Am J Physiol Endocrinol Metab 2013;304(12): E1314–20.

123. Alhadeff AL, Baird JP, Swick JC, et al. Glucagon-like Peptide-1 receptor signaling in the lateral parabrachial nucleus contributes to the control of food intake and motivation to feed. Neuropsychopharmacology 2014;39(9):2233–43.

124. Kastin AJ, Akerstrom V, Pan W. Interactions of glucagon-like peptide-1 (GLP-1) with the blood-brain barrier. J Mol Neurosci 2002;18(1–2):7–14.

125. Kanoski SE, Fortin SM, Arnold M, et al. Peripheral and Central GLP-1 Receptor Populations Mediate the Anorectic Effects of Peripherally Administered GLP-1 Receptor Agonists, Liraglutide and Exendin-4. Endocrinology 2011;152(8): 3103–12.

126. Tschop M, Smiley DL, Heiman ML. Ghrelin induces adiposity in rodents. Nature 2000;407(6806):908–13.

127. Wren AM, Small CJ, Ward HL, et al. The novel hypothalamic peptide ghrelin stimulates food intake and growth hormone secretion. Endocrinology 2000; 141(11):4325–8.

128. Cummings DE, Purnell JQ, Frayo RS, et al. A preprandial rise in plasma ghrelin levels suggests a role in meal initiation in humans. Diabetes 2001;50(8):1714–9.

129. Wren AM, Small CJ, Abbott CR, et al. Ghrelin causes hyperphagia and obesity in rats. Diabetes 2001;50(11):2540–7.

130. Asakawa A, Inui A, Kaga T, et al. Antagonism of ghrelin receptor reduces food intake and body weight gain in mice. Gut 2003;52(7):947–52.

131. Zigman JM, Jones JE, Lee CE, et al. Expression of ghrelin receptor mRNA in the rat and the mouse brain. J Comp Neurol 2006;494(3):528–48.

132. Kinzig KP, Scott KA, Hyun J, et al. Lateral ventricular ghrelin and fourth ventricular ghrelin induce similar increases in food intake and patterns of hypothalamic gene expression. Am J Physiol Regul Integr Comp Physiol 2006;290(6): R1565–9.

133. Shintani M, Ogawa Y, Ebihara K, et al. Ghrelin, an endogenous growth hormone secretagogue, is a novel orexigenic peptide that antagonizes leptin action through the activation of hypothalamic neuropeptide Y/Y1 receptor pathway. Diabetes 2001;50(2):227–32.

134. Seoane LM, López M, Tovar S, et al. Agouti-related peptide, neuropeptide Y, and somatostatin-producing neurons are targets for ghrelin actions in the rat hypothalamus. Endocrinology 2003;144(2):544–51.

135. Faulconbridge LF, Cummings DE, Kaplan JM, et al. Hyperphagic effects of brainstem ghrelin administration. Diabetes 2003;52(9):2260–5.

136. Zigman JM, Nakano Y, Coppari R, et al. Mice lacking ghrelin receptors resist the development of diet-induced obesity. J Clin Invest 2005;115(12):3564–72.

137. Wortley KE, Anderson KD, Garcia K, et al. Genetic deletion of ghrelin does not decrease food intake but influences metabolic fuel preference. Proc Natl Acad Sci U S A 2004;101(21):8227–32.

138. Pfluger PT, Kirchner H, Günnel S, et al. Simultaneous deletion of ghrelin and its receptor increases motor activity and energy expenditure. Am J Physiol Gastrointest Liver Physiol 2008;294(3):G610–8.

139. Cummings DE, Weigle DS, Frayo RS, et al. Plasma ghrelin levels after diet-induced weight loss or gastric bypass surgery. N Engl J Med 2002;346(21): 1623–30.

140. Gosnell BA, Krahn DD. The effects of continuous morphine infusion on diet selection and body weight. Physiol Behav 1993;54(5):853–9.

141. Doyle TG, Berridge KC, Gosnell BA. Morphine enhances hedonic taste palatability in rats. Pharmacol Biochem Behav 1993;46(3):745–9.

142. Glass MJ, Grace M, Cleary JP, et al. Potency of naloxone's anorectic effect in rats is dependent on diet preference. Am J Physiol 1996;271(1 Pt 2):R217–21.

143. Pecina S, Smith KS, Berridge KC. Hedonic hot spots in the brain. Neuroscientist 2006;12(6):500–11.

144. Pecina S, Berridge KC. Hedonic hot spot in nucleus accumbens shell: where do mu-opioids cause increased hedonic impact of sweetness? J Neurosci 2005; 25(50):11777–86.

145. Smith KS, Berridge KC. Opioid limbic circuit for reward: interaction between hedonic hotspots of nucleus accumbens and ventral pallidum. J Neurosci 2007; 27(7):1594–605.

146. Woolley JD, Lee BS, Taha SA, et al. Nucleus accumbens opioid signaling conditions short-term flavor preferences. Neuroscience 2007;146(1):19–30.

147. Sills TL, Vaccarino FJ. Facilitation and inhibition of feeding by a single dose of amphetamine: relationship to baseline intake and accumbens cholecystokinin. Psychopharmacology (Berl) 1991;105(3):329–34.

148. Ungerstedt U. Adipsia and aphagia after 6-hydroxydopamine induced degeneration of the nigro-striatal dopamine system. Acta Physiol Scand Suppl 1971;367: 95–122.

149. Zhou QY, Palmiter RD. Dopamine-deficient mice are severely hypoactive, adipsic, and aphagic. Cell 1995;83(7):1197–209.

150. Hernandez L, Hoebel BG. Feeding and hypothalamic stimulation increase dopamine turnover in the accumbens. Physiol Behav 1988;44(4–5):599–606.

151. Martel P, Fantino M. Mesolimbic dopaminergic system activity as a function of food reward: a microdialysis study. Pharmacol Biochem Behav 1996;53(1): 221–6.

152. Hajnal A, Smith GP, Norgren R. Oral sucrose stimulation increases accumbens dopamine in the rat. Am J Physiol Regul Integr Comp Physiol 2004;286(1): R31–7.

153. Liang NC, Hajnal A, Norgren R. Sham feeding corn oil increases accumbens dopamine in the rat. Am J Physiol Regul Integr Comp Physiol 2006;291(5): R1236–9.

154. Sclafani A, Ackroff K, Schwartz GJ. Selective effects of vagal deafferentation and celiac-superior mesenteric ganglionectomy on the reinforcing and satiating action of intestinal nutrients. Physiol Behav 2003;78(2):285–94.

155. Azzara AV, Bodnar RJ, Delamater AR, et al. Naltrexone fails to block the acquisition or expression of a flavor preference conditioned by intragastric carbohydrate infusions. Pharmacol Biochem Behav 2000;67(3):545–57.

156. Azzara AV, Bodnar RJ, Delamater AR, et al. D1 but not D2 dopamine receptor antagonism blocks the acquisition of a flavor preference conditioned by intragastric carbohydrate infusions. Pharmacol Biochem Behav 2001;68(4):709–20.

157. Bernal S, Miner P, Abayev Y, et al. Role of amygdala dopamine D1 and D2 receptors in the acquisition and expression of fructose-conditioned flavor preferences in rats. Behav Brain Res 2009;205(1):183–90.

158. de Araujo IE. Circuit organization of sugar reinforcement. Physiol Behav 2016; 164(Pt B):473–7.

159. Eckel LA, Langhans W, Kahler A, et al. Chronic administration of OB protein decreases food intake by selectively reducing meal size in female rats. Am J Physiol 1998;275(1 Pt 2):R186–93.

160. Kahler A, Geary N, Eckel L, et al. Chronic administration of OB protein decreases food intake by selectively reducing meal size in male rats. Am J Physiol 1998;275(1 Pt 2):R180–5.

161. Flynn MC, Scott TR, Pritchard TC, et al. Mode of action of OB protein (leptin) on feeding. Am J Physiol 1998;275(1 Pt 2):R174–9.

162. Barrachina MD, Martínez V, Wang L, et al. Synergistic interaction between leptin and cholecystokinin to reduce short-term food intake in lean mice. Proc Natl Acad Sci U S A 1997;94(19):10455–60.

163. Emond M, Schwartz GJ, Ladenheim EE, et al. Central leptin modulates behavioral and neural responsivity to CCK. Am J Physiol 1999;276(5 Pt 2):R1545–9.

164. Emond M, Ladenheim EE, Schwartz GJ, et al. Leptin amplifies the feeding inhibition and neural activation arising from a gastric nutrient preload. Physiol Behav 2001;72(1–2):123–8.

165. Schwartz GJ, Moran TH. Leptin and neuropeptide y have opposing modulatory effects on nucleus of the solitary tract neurophysiological responses to gastric loads: implications for the control of food intake. Endocrinology 2002;143(10): 3779–84.

166. McMinn JE, Sindelar DK, Havel PJ, et al. Leptin deficiency induced by fasting impairs the satiety response to cholecystokinin. Endocrinology 2000;141(12): 4442–8.

167. Moran TH, Aja S, Ladenheim EE. Leptin modulation of peripheral controls of meal size. Physiol Behav 2006;89(4):511–6.

168. Grill HJ, Schwartz MW, Kaplan JM, et al. Evidence that the caudal brainstem is a target for the inhibitory effect of leptin on food intake. Endocrinology 2002; 143(1):239–46.

169. Mahaut S, Dumont Y, Fournier A, et al. Neuropeptide Y receptor subtypes in the dorsal vagal complex under acute feeding adaptation in the adult rat. Neuropeptides 2010;44(2):77–86.

170. Figlewicz DP, Evans SB, Murphy J, et al. Expression of receptors for insulin and leptin in the ventral tegmental area/substantia nigra (VTA/SN) of the rat. Brain Res 2003;964(1):107–15.

171. Leininger GM, Jo YH, Leshan RL, et al. Leptin acts via leptin receptor-expressing lateral hypothalamic neurons to modulate the mesolimbic dopamine system and suppress feeding. Cell Metab 2009;10(2):89–98.

172. Fulton S, Woodside B, Shizgal P. Modulation of brain reward circuitry by leptin. Science 2000;287(5450):125–8.

173. Figlewicz DP, Bennett J, Evans SB, et al. Intraventricular insulin and leptin reverse place preference conditioned with high-fat diet in rats. Behav Neurosci 2004;118(3):479–87.

174. Perello M, Sakata I, Birnbaum S, et al. Ghrelin increases the rewarding value of high-fat diet in an orexin-dependent manner. Biol Psychiatry 2010;67(9):880–6.

175. Figlewicz DP. Adiposity signals and food reward: expanding the CNS roles of insulin and leptin. Am J Physiol Regul Integr Comp Physiol 2003;284(4): R882–92.
176. Matson CA, Reid DF, Cannon TA, et al. Cholecystokinin and leptin act synergistically to reduce body weight. Am J Physiol Regul Integr Comp Physiol 2000; 278(4):R882–90.
177. Matson CA, Wiater MF, Kuijper JL, et al. Synergy between leptin and cholecystokinin (CCK) to control daily caloric intake. Peptides 1997;18(8):1275–8.
178. Matson CA, Ritter RC. Long-term CCK-leptin synergy suggests a role for CCK in the regulation of body weight. Am J Physiol 1999;276(4 Pt 2):R1038–45.
179. Trevaskis JL, Coffey T, Cole R, et al. Amylin-mediated restoration of leptin responsiveness in diet-induced obesity: magnitude and mechanisms. Endocrinology 2008;149(11):5679–87.
180. Roth JD, Roland BL, Cole RL, et al. Leptin responsiveness restored by amylin agonism in diet-induced obesity: evidence from nonclinical and clinical studies. Proc Natl Acad Sci U S A 2008;105(20):7257–62.
181. Alhadeff AL, Rupprecht LE, Hayes MR. GLP-1 neurons in the nucleus of the solitary tract project directly to the ventral tegmental area and nucleus accumbens to control for food intake. Endocrinology 2012;153(2):647–58.
182. Mietlicki-Baase EG, Reiner DJ, Cone JJ, et al. Amylin modulates the mesolimbic dopamine system to control energy balance. Neuropsychopharmacology 2015; 40(2):372–85.
183. Baisley SK, Baldo BA. Amylin receptor signaling in the nucleus accumbens negatively modulates mu-opioid-driven feeding. Neuropsychopharmacology 2014;39(13):3009–17.
184. Will MJ, Franzblau EB, Kelley AE. Nucleus accumbens mu-opioids regulate intake of a high-fat diet via activation of a distributed brain network. J Neurosci 2003;23(7):2882–8.
185. Zheng H, Patterson LM, Berthoud HR. Orexin signaling in the ventral tegmental area is required for high-fat appetite induced by opioid stimulation of the nucleus accumbens. J Neurosci 2007;27(41):11075–82.
186. Zheng H, Townsend RL, Shin AC, et al. High-fat intake induced by mu-opioid activation of the nucleus accumbens is inhibited by Y1R-blockade and MC3/4R- stimulation. Brain Res 2010;1350:131–8.

The Gut Microbiota
The Gateway to Improved Metabolism

Kristina B. Martinez, PhD, RD[a], Joseph F. Pierre, PhD[a], Eugene B. Chang, MD[b],*

KEYWORDS

- Microbiota • Metabolism • Bariatric surgery • Enteroendocrine hormones
- Lipid absorption • Probiotics • Prebiotics • Synbiotics

KEY POINTS

- Shifts in the gut microbiome are inseparably associated with the development of obesity and comorbidities.
- Transfer of dysbiotic microbial communities confers disease phenotypes in recipients, supporting a central role for microbe-mediated regulation of metabolism.
- Bariatric surgery, the most effective treatment of morbid obesity, results in rapid changes in the gut microbiota, with concurrent improvements in metabolic parameters.
- Deeper understanding of host-microbe interactions may hold promise in the treatment of obesity, which remains a global epidemic.

INTRODUCTION: OBESITY AND THE GUT MICROBIOTA

The increase of obesity and its related comorbidities in westernized countries over the past 4 decades presents an emerging global epidemic with profound challenges to world health care economies and societies. In the past 35 years, the rate of adult obesity has risen by 75% globally.[1,2] This number is greater among children.[3,4] Stratified assessment of body mass index further shows disproportionate increases among the most severely obese ($\geq$35 kg/m^2), compared with the lesser obese ($\geq$30 kg/m^2), showing the scale of the problem. However, obesity and its comorbidities,[5] including metabolic syndrome, diabetes, and heart disease, have detrimental effects on quality of life and substantial costs to individuals and societies. Thus, the need for understanding the complexity of pathophysiologic events and elucidating effective interventions remain urgent.

Disclosure: This work was supported by NIH NIDDK DK42086 (DDRCC), DK097268, T32DK07074 to K.B. Martinez; F32DK105728-01A1 to J.F. Pierre.
[a] Section of Gastroenterology, Hepatology, and Nutrition, Department of Medicine, University of Chicago, Chicago, IL 60637, USA; [b] Section of Gastroenterology, Hepatology, and Nutrition, Department of Medicine, Knapp Center for Biomedical Discovery, University of Chicago, Room 9130, 900 East 57th Street, Chicago, IL 60637, USA
* Corresponding author.
E-mail address: echang@medicine.bsd.uchicago.edu

Gastroenterol Clin N Am 45 (2016) 601–614
http://dx.doi.org/10.1016/j.gtc.2016.07.001
0889-8553/16/© 2016 Elsevier Inc. All rights reserved.

The cause of obesity is multifactorial, including the complex interaction of genetics and environment, which encompasses diet, developmental factors, lifestyle (eg, hedonistic tendencies, altered sleep patterns), and antibiotic use. Intestinal microbes are affected by all of these factors in their community structure and function, and in turn initiate host-microbe interactions that may disrupt metabolic and immune homeostasis. Fecal microbiota transplant (FMT) of microbes under environmental stressors, like diet and obesity, can induce a similar phenotype in recipients.[6] The gut microbiome is by definition a microbial organ (vital to intestinal and systemic functions), and one that people cannot live without, but is also an organ that is transplantable (ie, via FMT). This technique is commonly used for *Clostridium difficile* infection and has only recently been studied for use in other conditions, including obesity. However, other therapies targeting the microbiome, such as prebiotics and probiotics, may confer modest, but positive, improvements for symptoms associated with obesity and its comorbidities.

Although an extreme measure reserved for the morbidly obese, one of the most effective strategies to decrease obesity is bariatric surgery, which profoundly changes the gut microbiota and energy balance, and alters physiologic and endocrine metabolic states.[7] It is expected that by changing metabolic set points, desired weight can be achieved. Therefore, understanding of the mechanisms behind bariatric surgery and associated changes in the gut microbiota may be leveraged to develop new therapies to fight the obesity epidemic. This article explores these concepts by providing an overview of altered microbial structure and function in obesity, host-microbe interactions driving obesity, dietary influence on the microbiome, improvements in metabolism and microbial structure with Roux-en-Y gastric bypass (RYGB), the host-microbe interactions driving obesity, and current therapies targeting the gut microbiome to facilitate positive metabolic outcomes.

PARADIGMS IN GUT MICROBIOTA DURING OBESITY
Obesity-Driven Alterations in Gut Microbiota

The human body contains huge numbers of microbes, including thousands of bacterial species, in addition to many eukaryotes, Achaea, protists, and viruses, which collectively contain an estimated 5 million genes that have profound metabolic and immunomodulatory effects on their mammalian hosts.[8] The community of microbes is termed the microbiota, whereas their collective genes are called the microbiome. Both the state of obesity and westernized diets are associated with microbial dysbiosis, which is a deviation from microbial organization that would otherwise promote optimal metabolic homeostasis. Dysbiotic microbiota in obesity is characterized by decreased diversity in the microbial community and by an increased ratio of the phylum Firmicutes to the phylum Bacteroidetes.[9] The change in the Firmicutes/Bacteroidetes ratio occurs in both mice and humans, and weight loss restores microbial composition.[9–11] Note that 3 genera of bacteria are often overrepresented in obesity in humans: *Bacteroides* and *Prevotella* (both Bacteroidetes) and *Ruminococcus* (Firmicutes).[12] In addition to composition, major functional differences are observed in metabolic capacity of the microbial community. For instance, decreases in short-chain fatty acid (SCFA) producers, such as from the phylum Actinobacteria and blooms in pathogenic bacteria from the phylum Proteobacteria, occur in obesity.[13] In addition to bacteria, recent work shows that the microbiota metabolic networks include yeast and archaea, which synergistically produce and use metabolites collectively with bacteria.[14] Although this area is still underexplored, recent work suggests that yeast species abundance is lower in obesity, and supplementation with *Saccharomyces cerevisiae* improves metabolic parameters and adiposity.[15–17]

When dysbiotic communities of bacteria are transferred to naive germ-free (GF) mice, the recipient mice develop increased adiposity, showing a direct impact of the microbes on advancing fat storage in the mammalian host.[6] Although some bacteria are associated with excess adiposity, others have been directly implicated in improving metabolic syndrome and atherosclerosis, such as *Akkermansia muciniphila*,[18,19] and are often found to be underrepresented in obesity. Administration of *A muciniphila* during obesity was shown to improve glucose tolerance.[19] Schneeberger and colleagues[18] found that among 27 genes that regulate inflammation and metabolism in white adipose tissue under high-fat feeding, 20 genes negatively correlate with the relative abundance of *A muciniphila*. In addition, *Bifidobacterium* spp also negatively correlated with 6 of 27 genes. Positive correlations were observed with *Bilophila wadsworthia* in 14 of 27 genes, and this microbe is known to expand under high-milk-fat diets and subsequently stimulate inflammatory responses.[20] Together these observations suggest that certain microbes might regulate aspects of peripheral metabolism related to obesity and metabolism, but further investigations to determine strong proof of causality are required.

Another line of evidence that supports the notion that microbes might closely regulate host metabolism and body weight is found through the study of acute malnutrition in childhood. In contrast with overfed and obese individuals, work by Subramanian and colleagues[21] followed severely malnourished children for 2 years. Through compositional modeling, they showed that the microbiota normally develop with growing children, but, with malnutrition, the microbiota maturity remains stunted and lags behind host development. Even after common therapeutic food interventions, the immaturity of the microbiota persisted. Note that the microbiota remains immature even under less severe malnourished states and that microbiota maturity correlated with anthropometric measurements of the children.[21] These findings strongly support the notion of the gut microbiota functioning as a vital organ, and its development and growth throughout life may have important unknown implications for human health. Understanding the role of microbial development under states of hyperalimentation may provide insights into dysfunctional microbial-host metabolic interactions that lead to excessive fat storage.

Dietary Impact on the Gut Microbiota

Although host phenotype influences the composition of the microbial communities, diet also notably has an immediate and dramatic impact on microbial structure that mimics communities seen in obese individuals. For instance, David and colleagues[22] observed in humans that a diet rich in animal-derived fat and protein resulted in significant changes in the gut microbiota in as little as a day, and, of particular note, blooms in hydrogen sulfide–producing bacteria such as *B wadsworthia* were also observed. Later, his group found that diet has a greater impact on altering microbial assemblage than genetic background in mice.[23] In this study, 5 different inbred mouse strains, 4 genetic knockout strains relevant to host-microbe interactions (eg, ob/ob, NOD2, MyD88−/−, and Rag1−/−), and 200 outbred mice were placed on high-fat, high-sugar diets or diets rich in plant polysaccharides. In each experiment, the Western diet had profoundly altered community structure, regardless of strain differences or gene deficiencies.[23] More recently, Sonnenburg and colleagues[24] showed that diets low in microbe-accessible carbohydrate (MAC) and high in simple sugars result in loss of bacterial diversity and extinction of specific microbial groups that is compounded over generations. The generational loss of bacterial diversity could only be remedied with FMT from control mice maintained on the MAC-rich diet, but not by diet alone. This study provides a model for the rapid and drastic impact of the human food supply, containing readily available processed high-fat and high-sugar food, on the progressive loss of bacterial diversity over the past several decades. This theory postulates that human bodies are not equipped to reciprocate and adapt to the sudden insult on the gut microbiota, thereby leading to the development of obesity. Based on the results from this study, suitable therapies to combat the loss of bacterial diversity might include probiotic supplementation or FMT.

High-fat diets also transform the metagenomes of the bacteriophage community, also known as the phageome. It was shown by Howe and colleagues[25] that high-fat diets can shift the phageome independent of observed alterations in the bacterial host pattern. The impact of diet on viral communities was also rapid, occurring within 24 hours. In addition, the change in the viral metagenomes by the high-fat diet was not reversible after washout, suggesting that diet-mediated changes in the phage community are persistent, similar to the aforementioned findings in bacteria.[25] Further research in this area is needed to better understand the regulation and function of the phageome, its impact on gut microbial ecology, and more importantly consequences for the host.

Restructuring of Gut Microbiota in Bariatric Surgery

Surgical intervention, although largely invasive, is the most effective weight loss strategy for obesity. RYGB is the most common and the most effective, promoting a 20% to 40% weight loss compared with 15% to 30% loss of body weight with gastric banding.[26] RYGB includes the formation of a small pouch, made of the upper stomach, that is then attached to a region of jejunum approximately 75 cm distal to the stomach (termed a gastrojejunostomy). The resulting limb (including the distal stomach) carries bile, gastric juice, and pancreatic juices alone, without nutrients, another 125 cm distal from the gastrojejunostomy, collectively delaying the mixture of digestive juices and nutrients for approximately 200 cm of the upper gastrointestinal (GI) tract. It is becoming increasingly apparent that bariatric surgery, particularly RYGB, may involve multiple mechanisms beyond simple physical restrictions to nutrient intake and absorption through reduced stomach size and decreased absorptive capacity. It is plausible that new treatments will be discovered based on the mechanisms underlying bariatric surgery efficaciousness. Intriguing data suggest that the mechanisms involved may include altered gut microbial function[7] and interactions of the microbiome with the host's bile acid pool.[27,28]

Anatomic rearrangement triggers the dramatic restructuring of the intestinal microbiota and host-microbe interactions that may contribute to weight loss after bariatric surgery. For example, RYGB in mice resulted in the rapid restructuring of gut microbiota as early as 1 week compared with sham controls.[7] The early changes in microbial composition occur within the same time frames as improvement in glucose tolerance and reduced insulin resistance,[29] in contrast with body weight and adiposity changes that occur over weeks and months, suggesting that microbial alterations may be involved in the resetting of metabolic set points that are distinct from adiposity. Specifically, RYGB results in a decrease in the Firmicutes/Bacteroidetes ratio, which includes increases in Bacteroidales, Enterobacteriales, as well as increases in Gammaproteobacteria (*Escherichia coli*) and Verrucomicrobia[7] as a relative percentage of the microbial community. Note that the Verrucomicrobia genus *Akkermansia* uses host secretion of mucin as a fuel source and has been inversely correlated with body weight.[19] As previously discussed, oral administration of live *A muciniphila* restores insulin sensitivity in high-fat fed animals.[19] Following RYGB in diabetic rodents, the level of *A muciniphila* in the small bowel increased significantly compared with sham obese controls.[30] The increase in *A muciniphila* was positively related with the release of GLP-1, an important intestinal incretin, suggesting that this microbe could be modulating peripheral glucose handling through modulated insulin tolerance. In humans following RYGB, an inverse correlation in the relative percentages of E coli, Bacteroides, and Prevotella with circulating leptin levels was found, an important adipose factor released at higher levels in obesity.[31] In addition, the increases in Proteobacteria observed following RYGB have reached 50-fold, and together with other models suggest that Proteobacteria may influence insulin sensitivity.[32,33] A direct role for the microbial community in mediating host metabolism following RYGB was confirmed with FMT from bariatric surgery donors into recipients, which conferred protection from obesity.[34] Altogether, these studies provide strong evidence that the gut microbiota may significantly contribute to the effectiveness of RYGB surgery, paving the way for focused investigations into altering the microbiota in a similar manner for the treatment of obesity.

The direct role for microbes in improving metabolism following RYGB remains under investigation, but other indirect roles include microbial changes to the bile acid composition; bile acid activation of the ileal and colonic bile acid receptors; and regulation of gut peptide enteroendocrine hormones, such as GLP-1 and peptide tyrosine tyrosine (PYY). Current evidence suggests that the composition of bile acids influences the microbiota assemblage through antimicrobial function,[27,28] because bile acids are detergents and influence the membrane chemistry. Reciprocally, bacteria influence bile acid composition by deconjugation and fermentation of primary bile acids into secondary and tertiary bile acids, which have differential effects on host metabolism. Primary bile acids are associated with improved metabolism, whereas secondary bile acids are potentially carcinogenic and not associated with metabolic improvement.[35,36] Therefore, bile acids and microbial compositions are inseparably associated and continually interacting in the gut. Novel work showed that bile acid–altered microbial communities in turn influence host metabolism, establishing a crosstalk between bile acids and the intestinal microbiome that influences host metabolism.[37] In addition to altering bacterial viability and growth, and aiding in the absorption of luminal dietary lipids and lipid vitamins, bile acids directly modulate host metabolism through host bile acid receptors.[27,38] Bile acid interactions with the G protein–coupled bile acid receptor 1 (GPBAR1 or TGR5) and farnesoid X receptor (FXR) regulate peripheral energy expenditure and counteract obesity and diabetes. On activation by bile acids, TGR5 specifically stimulates the release of GLP-1, GLP-2, and PYY from enteroendocrine cells as well as expression of various transport proteins and biosynthetics, resulting in improved glycemic control. Enteroendocrine cells also contain toll-like receptors and sense bacteria in the intestinal lumen.[39] Following RYGB, increased circulating levels of GLP-1 and PYY are reported.[40,41] PYY is normally released postprandially to increase energy expenditure and decrease food intake. In healthy individuals, PYY release following feeding is proportionate to caloric consumption, acting directly on the hypothalamus and vagal afferents to slow feeding behavior.[42] It remains unclear whether increased PYY and GLP-1 levels following RYGB are in response to altered microbial populations, bile acid pools, or a combination. Regardless, changes in intestinal enteroendocrine signaling following RYGB have profound effects on host metabolism and multiple lines of evidence now strongly support the involvement of the microbiota.

HOST-MICROBE INTERACTIONS DRIVING OBESITY

The observation that GF mice are resistant to diet-induced obesity has created a foundation for understanding the contribution of microbes and host-microbe interactions to the development of obesity and its comorbidities. Several mechanisms to explain microbe-mediated obesity have been proposed, including (1) SCFA production; (2) regulation of food intake and sensory perception of food; (3) nutrient absorption; (4) circulation of microbe-derived enterotoxins like lipopolysaccharides (LPS) and reduced production of angiopoietinlike 4 (angptl4), resulting in increased fatty acid uptake in liver and adipose tissue[13]; and (5) peripheral control of circadian rhythm, which is intimately linked to metabolic coordination between the brain and peripheral organs.[43,44]

One metabolic function of microbes is the production of SCFAs, including acetate, propionate, and butyrate, from otherwise indigestible fibers. SCFAs can act as energy sources for the intestinal epithelium and liver, and mouse models of obesity show increased SCFA in luminal content and lower energy content in feces.[45] However, SCFAs have many reported beneficial effects on metabolism and improved glucose tolerance. For instance, diets supplemented with fructo-oligosaccharides (FOSs), butyrate, and propionate decreased weight gain and improved glucose tolerance in rats compared with controls. It was shown that these positive effects were mediated through stimulation of intestinal gluconeogenesis, because mice deficient in the catalytic subunit of glucose-6 phosphatase displayed impaired glucose tolerance.[46] Thus, conflicting evidence exists regarding the negative consequences of increased energy availability through SCFA production given the potential positive impact of SCFAs on metabolism.

Obesity is also related to peripheral inflammation, especially in adipose tissue. The gut microbiota influences gut permeability, which may lead to entry of microbial ligands, including LPS, into the blood stream and periphery, where they can induce insulin resistance and prevent peripheral uptake of fat.[47–49] Intriguingly, bioactive dietary components such as omega 3 fatty acids and polyphenols that are reported to improve adipose inflammation also affect microbial structure. For example, Backhed's group showed that the gut microbiota exacerbates adipose inflammation through toll-like receptor signaling on saturated fat feeding, as has been suspected for some time in adipose biology.[50] Notably, microbiota transplant from fish oil–fed mice attenuated weight gain in antibiotic mice that were maintained on a lard diet.[50] Cranberry and grape polyphenols have also been reported to alter microbial structure, specifically via increasing the abundance of *A muciniphila*, as well as improving glucose tolerance and adipose inflammation.[51,52]

Microbial regulation of metabolism is mediated in part through the sensory perception of food, GI motility, and nutrient absorption, because these are altered in GF mice. For instance, GF mice have increased preference for sugar-sweetened liquids and fat emulsions but lack the machinery to process the nutrients. Swartz and colleagues[53] found that GF mice consume more sucrose solution concurrent with increased expression of type 1 taste receptor 3 (TIR3) expression and sodium glucose luminal transporter 1 (SGLT1) in the small intestinal epithelium compared with conventional mice.[53] Anorexigenic gut peptide hormones, including PYY and cholesytokinin (CCK), are also regulated by gut microbes facilitating control of food intake. Although GF mice have increased expression of lingual fatty acid translocase (CD36), expression of gut peptide hormones, including PYY, CCK, and GLP-1, was reduced in the intestinal epithelium, as well as decreased numbers of enteroendocrine cells (EECs) in the ileum.[54] In contrast with these gut peptide hormones, Backhed's group reported that GF mice have increased levels of GLP-1, which slows gastric motility and increases intestinal transit time as a compensatory mechanism to allow enhanced nutrient absorption.[55] Given the role of enteroendocrine hormone signaling in nutrient absorption, dysregulation of these hormones may explain why GF mice have increased levels of triglycerides and total lipids in their stool after high-fat diet feeding.[56] In addition, conventionalization of GF zebrafish increases lipid accumulation in the intestinal epithelium.[43] Taken together, these findings suggest that gut microbes facilitate hormonal cues to regulate sensory perception of food, dietary intake, as well as nutrient absorption. However, the exact mechanisms behind microbial regulation of carbohydrate and lipid absorption and the extent to which microbe-induced nutrient absorption significantly contributes to obesity have not been well characterized.

Differences between GF and conventional mice also involve dysregulation of bile production. Because of the lack of microbes in GF mice, there is little to no deconjugation of conjugated bile acids entering the GI lumen, thereby resulting in high levels of taurine-conjugated bile acids in GF mice compared with conventional mice.[37] Backhed's group reported that increased taurine-conjugated bile acids block FXR-mediated induction of fibroblast growth factor 15 (FGF-15), which would otherwise decrease bile acid synthesis in the liver. Thus, GF mice have increased bile acid production. This study implicates the role of gut microbiota in regulating bile acid metabolism through a gut-liver axis.[57]

The difference in bile acid metabolism speaks to the marked difference in liver function between GF and conventional mice. GF mice have decreased liver lipid content and altered expression of gene networks, including those involving xenobiotic metabolism and circadian rhythm.[58] At the hub of xenobiotic gene networks are 2 nuclear hormone receptors, constitutive androstane receptor (CAR) and pregnane X receptor (PXR), which are implicated in regulating whole-body metabolism. Activation of CAR has been shown to decrease body weight and improve insulin sensitivity, whereas PXR activation has been positively associated with obesity.[59–61] Thus, it is tempting to speculate that CAR-mediated metabolic activity in GF mice may contribute to their resistance to high-fat diet–induced obesity. However, this connection has not been thoroughly investigated in the current literature.

Gut microbes have been found to control circadian function. This finding has important implications for fighting obesity, because the disruption of the natural cycle of day and night (eg, jet lag, shift work, and sleep apnea) contributes to the increasing prevalence of metabolic disorders.[13] Circadian rhythms are regulated by molecular clocks that coordinate regularly timed events (ie, states of feeding vs fasting) and the necessary physiologic responses to enhance metabolic efficiency. Thus, circadian rhythm is intimately linked to the regulation of food intake, activity, and whole-body metabolism involving clocks located in the brain as well as peripheral metabolic tissues. The circadian transcriptional program is under the control of 2 major transcriptional activators, Bmal and Clock, which are counter-regulated by repressors, Period 1 to 3 and Cryptochrome 1 and 2. Consumption of high-fat diets represses diurnal variation of these gene transcripts and impairs normal circadian function.[62] It has recently been shown that these changes depend on the gut microbiota, because GF mice and antibiotic-treated mice have reduced expression of Bmal and Clock and increased expression of Period 1 to 3, and Cryptochrome 1 and 2 in the intestinal epithelium.[63] It was later shown by Leone and colleagues[44] that diurnal variation in the circadian gene program is also blunted in the liver of GF compared with specific pathogen free (SPF) mice.

In addition to host circadian rhythm, microbes display circadian behavior.[44] Strikingly, community structure of the gut microbiota as well as butyrate shows diurnal variation over a 24-hour period under normal feeding conditions and is diminished under high-fat feeding. To ensure that these changes were not caused by times of feeding, stool was collected from mice on total parenteral nutrition (TPN) and compared with mice fed enterally. Although differences existed in the relative abundance of specific microbes (eg, increase in Verrucomicrobia in the TPN group), diurnal shifts were still evident, indicating that microbial abundance may fluctuate based on host cues, such as the release of mucin or other epithelial proteins and secretions. Altogether these findings suggest that the regulation of host circadian function depends on the activity of the gut microbiota and, conversely, the circadian behavior of the gut microbiota depends on host physiology.[13,44] Identifying the host-microbe interactions that facilitate microbial control of circadian rhythm may lead to therapies targeting the gut microbiota to restore the metabolic consequences of disrupted sleep, which is common in obesity.

TREATMENTS TARGETING MICROBIOME TO FIGHT OBESITY AND METABOLIC SYNDROME

The host-microbiome field is moving toward improving metabolism and weight maintenance through modulating gut microbial communities using a variety of supplements such as prebiotics and probiotics, synbiotics, FMT, and postbiotics. Prebiotics are foods or dietary supplements that encourage the growth of saccharolytic bacteria that metabolize nondigestible carbohydrates such as inulin and oligofructose. Several criteria must be met for a supplement to be considered a prebiotic and these include resistance to gastric acidity, nondigestible by the host in the small intestine, bacterial fermentation, and promotion of beneficial bacteria.[64]

Prebiotics

Prebiotics have recently been shown to improve complications associated with metabolic disorders, including obesity and insulin resistance.[65] Various mechanisms have been identified to explain these beneficial effects, including SCFA production, stimulation of intestinal gluconeogenesis, epithelial integrity, release of hormones PYY and GLP1 to promote satiety and insulin sensitivity, increased expression of antimicrobial peptides, and alteration of gut microbial community structure.[65]

Gene expression of the antimicrobial peptide, Reg3y, was reduced after high-fat diet feeding but restored on delivery of oligofructose.[34] Prebiotic supplementation also increased intectin expression, which promotes epithelial cell turnover and maintenance. FOS treatment in mice fed a Western diet improved glucose and insulin tolerance compared with controls. The therapeutic effect of FOS was lost in mice deficient in glucose-6-phosphatase catalytic subunit, thereby shutting down intestinal gluconeogenesis. These findings suggest that intestinal gluconeogenesis is necessary for FOS-mediated glucose and insulin sensitivity.[46] Similar results have been shown in humans. For example, participants fed brown beans[66] or prebiotics containing wheat fiber and soluble fiber[67] showed improved insulin sensitivity. Taken together, these findings support the use of prebiotic therapy in both animals and humans for improved metabolic health.

Probiotics

Another commonly used approach and widely studied supplement is the use of probiotics, which are live microorganisms delivered individually or in combinations, such as VSL#3, that produce positive health outcomes in the host.[64] It is important to consider the composition of probiotic formulations because each strain may have a different impact; for example, on microbial structure/function or on the host immune response. Wang and colleagues[65] showed in mice that 3 strains of bacteria (*Lactobacillus paracasei* CNCM I-4270, *Lactobacillus rhamnosus* I-3690, and *Bifidobacterium animalis* subspecies *lactis* I-2494) independently decreased body weight and improved glucose tolerance but through different mechanisms (reviewed in Ref.[13]). Daily gavage of the probiotic yeast *Saccharomyces boulardii* (Biocodex) elicited changes in gut microbiota, reflecting a less obesogenic state, as well as improving the metabolic profile of genetically obese and diabetic db/db mice.[17]

A common concern with probiotics use is the lack of colonization following supplementation.[68] In addition, mixed-strain probiotics like VSL#3 or a symbiotic, which is the combination of a probiotic and prebiotic, may be more effective than single microbial isolates alone. VSL#3 contains 7 different strains belonging to the genera *Bifidobacterium* and *Lactobacillus* and has been shown to improve nonalcoholic fatty liver disease in children[69] and reduce the risk of hepatic encephalopathy in patients with cirrhosis.[70] Because of the complexity in formulating probiotic and prebiotic supplements, more research is needed to maximize their effectiveness for ameliorating metabolic disorders associated with obesity.

Fecal Microbiota Transplant

Other alternative therapies include FMT and postbiotics. FMT is the transfer of fecal slurries to a recipient from an approved donor. Although FMT is effective in ~90% cases of *C difficile* infection,[71] its use for other diseases in humans is still under investigation. Intriguingly, FMT from bariatric patients results in an improved metabolic profile in mice.[72] However, few reports exist for the use of FMT in relation to metabolic disease. However, it was shown by Vrieze and colleagues[73] that FMT improved symptoms related to insulin resistance in men with metabolic syndrome. Along with further study for metabolic disease, well-defined safety practices are needed for the use of FMT (reviewed in Ref.[74]).

Postbiotics

More recently, research has focused largely on metabolomics and the introduction of postbiotics, which are new formulations containing purified microbial metabolites or bacterial components that have a defined benefit to the host, as opposed to live bacteria in probiotics. Postbiotics may become a popular treatment option, because this targeted approach involves small, bioactive molecules that have a defined and specific function, without the potential adverse side effects that live bacteria may promote. For example, ex vivo culture with the probiotic *Lactobacillus plantarum* NCIMB8826 elicited an undesired immune response, but the culture media protected against *Salmonella*-mediated tumor necrosis factor secretion from intestinal mucosal explants.[75] The use of postbiotics would bypass adverse effects promoted by unknown processes triggered by probiotic formulations or potential pathogens delivered via FMT.

SUMMARY

Obesity and metabolic disease have various underlying causes, including genetics and environmental factors, making appropriate and effective treatments difficult to identify. The emergence of high-throughput sequencing has recently made it possible to examine the intestinal microbiome in the context of obesity. Understanding how the microbiota structure and function changes in states of obesity as well as bariatric surgery may resolve the role of the microbiome in regulating host metabolic set points, likely including interactions with the endocrine and nervous systems. The use of 16s ribosomal RNA amplicon sequencing is now routinely performed by many laboratories, but offers only limited information regarding the microbial members present under certain conditions, such as obesity, malnutrition, and RYGB surgery. It does not provide information regarding the function of key microbial species that drive host outcomes. Without this information it is difficult to determine which strains to examine for potentially vital host-microbe interactions. The complex and individualized nature of obesity presents another obstacle in understanding how clinicians can use the microbial organ. Which organ and what pathways should be targeted and how do clinicians determine this on an individual basis? However, with further advances and use of available technologies, such as metagenomics and metabolomics, keystone microbes should be better identified and interaction with the host understood, which will allow the creation of a database of potential pathobionts to target in order to modulate the microbial community. In contrast, these techniques can also be applied to beneficial microbes to understand how they can be used for developing more effective prebiotic, probiotic, or postbiotic therapies.

REFERENCES

1. Flegal KM. Epidemiologic aspects of overweight and obesity in the United States. Physiol Behav 2005;86(5):599–602.
2. Sturm R, Hattori A. Morbid obesity rates continue to rise rapidly in the United States. Int J Obes (Lond) 2013;37(6):889–91.
3. Bray GA. Obesity: a time bomb to be defused. Lancet 1998;352(9123):160–1.
4. de Onis M, Blossner M, Borghi E. Global prevalence and trends of overweight and obesity among preschool children. Am J Clin Nutr 2010;92(5):1257–64.
5. Ogden CL, Carroll MD, Curtin LR, et al. Prevalence of overweight and obesity in the United States, 1999-2004. JAMA 2006;295(13):1549–55.
6. Turnbaugh PJ, Ridaura VK, Faith JJ, et al. The effect of diet on the human gut microbiome: a metagenomic analysis in humanized gnotobiotic mice. Sci Transl Med 2009;1(6):6ra14.
7. Liou AP, Paziuk M, Luevano J-M, et al. Conserved shifts in the gut microbiota due to gastric bypass reduce host weight and adiposity. Sci Transl Med 2013;5(178): 178ra41.
8. Amar J, Serino M, Lange C, et al. Involvement of tissue bacteria in the onset of diabetes in humans: evidence for a concept. Diabetologia 2011;54(12):3055–61.
9. Ley RE, Bäckhed F, Turnbaugh P, et al. Obesity alters gut microbial ecology. Proc Natl Acad Sci U S A 2005;102(31):11070–5.
10. Shen W, Gaskins HR, McIntosh MK. Influence of dietary fat on intestinal microbes, inflammation, barrier function and metabolic outcomes. J Nutr Biochem 2014; 25(3):270–80.
11. Ley RE, Turnbaugh PJ, Klein S, et al. Microbial ecology: human gut microbes associated with obesity. Nature 2006;444(7122):1022–3.
12. Gill SR, Pop M, Deboy RT, et al. Metagenomic analysis of the human distal gut microbiome. Science 2006;312(5778):1355–9.
13. Ojeda P, Bobe A, Dolan K, et al. Nutritional modulation of gut microbiota - the impact on metabolic disease pathophysiology. J Nutr Biochem 2016;28:191–200.
14. Hoffmann C, Dollive S, Grunberg S, et al. Archaea and fungi of the human gut microbiome: correlations with diet and bacterial residents. PLoS One 2013;8(6): e66019.
15. Borgo F, Verduci E, Riva A, et al. Relative abundance in bacterial and fungal gut microbes in obese children: a case control study. Child Obes 2016. [Epub ahead of print].
16. de Araújo TV, Andrade EF, Lobato RV, et al. Effects of beta-glucans ingestion (*Saccharomyces cerevisiae*) on metabolism of rats receiving high-fat diet. J Anim Physiol Anim Nutr (Berl) 2016. http://dx.doi.org/10.1111/jpn.12452.

17. Everard A, Matamoros S, Geurts L, et al. *Saccharomyces boulardii* administration changes gut microbiota and reduces hepatic steatosis, low-grade inflammation, and fat mass in obese and type 2 diabetic db/db mice. MBio 2014;5(3): e01011–4.

18. Schneeberger M, Everard A, Gómez-Valadés AG, et al. *Akkermansia muciniphila* inversely correlates with the onset of inflammation, altered adipose tissue metabolism and metabolic disorders during obesity in mice. Sci Rep 2015;5:16643.

19. Everard A, Belzer C, Geurts L, et al. Cross-talk between *Akkermansia muciniphila* and intestinal epithelium controls diet-induced obesity. Proc Natl Acad Sci U S A 2013;110(22):9066–71.

20. Devkota S, Wang Y, Musch MW, et al. Dietary-fat-induced taurocholic acid promotes pathobiont expansion and colitis in Il10-/- mice. Nature 2012;487(7405): 104–8.

21. Subramanian S, Huq S, Yatsunenko T, et al. Persistent gut microbiota immaturity in malnourished Bangladeshi children. Nature 2014;510(7505):417–21.

22. David LA, Maurice CF, Carmody RN, et al. Diet rapidly and reproducibly alters the human gut microbiome. Nature 2014;505(7484):559–63.

23. Carmody RN, Gerber GK, Luevano JM Jr, et al. Diet dominates host genotype in shaping the murine gut microbiota. Cell Host Microbe 2015;17(1):72–84.

24. Sonnenburg ED, Smits SA, Tikhonov M, et al. Diet-induced extinctions in the gut microbiota compound over generations. Nature 2016;529(7585):212–5.

25. Howe A, Ringus DL, Williams RJ, et al. Divergent responses of viral and bacterial communities in the gut microbiome to dietary disturbances in mice. ISME J 2016; 10(5):1217–27.

26. Tadross JA, le Roux CW. The mechanisms of weight loss after bariatric surgery. Int J Obes (Lond) 2009;33(Suppl 1):S28–32.

27. Islam KB, Fukiya S, Hagio M, et al. Bile acid is a host factor that regulates the composition of the cecal microbiota in rats. Gastroenterology 2011;141(5): 1773–81.

28. Begley M, Gahan CG, Hill C. The interaction between bacteria and bile. FEMS Microbiol Rev 2005;29(4):625–51.

29. Kashyap SR, Daud S, Kelly KR, et al. Acute effects of gastric bypass versus gastric restrictive surgery on beta-cell function and insulinotropic hormones in severely obese patients with type 2 diabetes. Int J Obes (Lond) 2010;34(3): 462–71.

30. Yan M, Song MM, Bai RX, et al. Effect of Roux-en-Y gastric bypass surgery on intestinal *Akkermansia muciniphila*. World J Gastrointest Surg 2016;8(4):301–7.

31. Furet JP, Kong LC, Tap J, et al. Differential adaptation of human gut microbiota to bariatric surgery-induced weight loss: links with metabolic and low-grade inflammation markers. Diabetes 2010;59(12):3049–57.

32. Zhang H, DiBaise JK, Zuccolo A, et al. Human gut microbiota in obesity and after gastric bypass. Proc Natl Acad Sci U S A 2009;106(7):2365–70.

33. Carvalho BM, Guadagnini D, Tsukumo DM, et al. Modulation of gut microbiota by antibiotics improves insulin signalling in high-fat fed mice. Diabetologia 2012; 55(10):2823–34.

34. Everard A, Lazarevic V, Gaïa N, et al. Microbiome of prebiotic-treated mice reveals novel targets involved in host response during obesity. ISME J 2014; 8(10):2116–30.

35. Baptissart M, Vega A, Maqdasy S, et al. Bile acids: from digestion to cancers. Biochimie 2013;95(3):504–17.

36. Watanabe M, Houten SM, Mataki C, et al. Bile acids induce energy expenditure by promoting intracellular thyroid hormone activation. Nature 2006;439(7075): 484–9.

37. Swann JR, Want EJ, Geier FM, et al. Systemic gut microbial modulation of bile acid metabolism in host tissue compartments. Proc Natl Acad Sci U S A 2011; 108(Suppl 1):4523–30.

38. Inagaki T, Moschetta A, Lee YK, et al. Regulation of antibacterial defense in the small intestine by the nuclear bile acid receptor. Proc Natl Acad Sci U S A 2006;103(10):3920–5.

39. Palazzo M, Balsari A, Rossini A, et al. Activation of enteroendocrine cells via TLRs induces hormone, chemokine, and defensin secretion. J Immunol 2007;178(7): 4296–303. Available at: http://www.ncbi.nlm.nih.gov/pubmed/17371986. Accessed May 26, 2016.

40. Dirksen C, Jørgensen NB, Bojsen-Møller KN, et al. Gut hormones, early dumping and resting energy expenditure in patients with good and poor weight loss response after Roux-en-Y gastric bypass. Int J Obes (Lond) 2013;37(11):1452–9.

41. le Roux CW, Borg C, Wallis K, et al. Gut hypertrophy after gastric bypass is associated with increased glucagon-like peptide 2 and intestinal crypt cell proliferation. Ann Surg 2010;252(1):50–6.

42. Batterham RL, Cowley MA, Small CJ, et al. Gut hormone PYY(3-36) physiologically inhibits food intake. Nature 2002;418(6898):650–4.

43. Semova I, Carten JD, Stombaugh J, et al. Microbiota regulate intestinal absorption and metabolism of fatty acids in the zebrafish. Cell Host Microbe 2012;12(3): 277–88.

44. Leone V, Gibbons SM, Martinez K, et al. Effects of diurnal variation of gut microbes and high-fat feeding on host circadian clock function and metabolism. Cell Host Microbe 2015;17(5):681–9.

45. Schwiertz A, Taras D, Schäfer K, et al. Microbiota and SCFA in lean and overweight healthy subjects. Obesity 2010;18(1):190–5.

46. De Vadder F, Kovatcheva-Datchary P, Goncalves D, et al. Microbiota-generated metabolites promote metabolic benefits via gut-brain neural circuits. Cell 2014; 156(1–2):84–96.

47. Karlsson FH, Tremaroli V, Nookaew I, et al. Gut metagenome in European women with normal, impaired and diabetic glucose control. Nature 2013;498(7452): 99–103.

48. Karastergiou K, Fried SK, Xie H, et al. Distinct developmental signatures of human abdominal and gluteal subcutaneous adipose tissue depots. J Clin Endocrinol Metab 2013;98(1):362–71.

49. Cani PD, Delzenne NM. Gut microflora as a target for energy and metabolic homeostasis. Curr Opin Clin Nutr Metab Care 2007;10(6):729–34.

50. Caesar R, Tremaroli V, Kovatcheva-Datchary P, et al. Crosstalk between gut microbiota and dietary lipids aggravates wat inflammation through TLR signaling. Cell Metab 2015;22(4):658–68.

51. Anhê FF, Roy D, Pilon G, et al. A polyphenol-rich cranberry extract protects from diet-induced obesity, insulin resistance and intestinal inflammation in association with increased *Akkermansia* spp. population in the gut microbiota of mice. Gut 2015;64(6):872–83.

52. Collins B, Hoffman J, Martinez K, et al. A polyphenol-rich fraction obtained from table grapes decreases adiposity, insulin resistance and markers of inflammation and impacts gut microbiota in high-fat-fed mice. J Nutr Biochem 2016;31:150–65.

53. Swartz TD, Duca FA, de Wouters T, et al. Up-regulation of intestinal type 1 taste receptor 3 and sodium glucose luminal transporter-1 expression and increased sucrose intake in mice lacking gut microbiota. Br J Nutr 2012;107(5):621–30.
54. Duca FA, Swartz TD, Sakar Y, et al. Increased oral detection, but decreased intestinal signaling for fats in mice lacking gut microbiota. PLoS One 2012;7(6): e39748.
55. Wichmann A, Allahyar A, Greiner TU, et al. Microbial modulation of energy availability in the colon regulates intestinal transit. Cell Host Microbe 2013;14(5): 582–90.
56. Rabot S, Membrez M, Bruneau A, et al. Germ-free C57BL/6J mice are resistant to high-fat-diet-induced insulin resistance and have altered cholesterol metabolism. FASEB J 2010;24(12):4948–59.
57. Sayin SI, Wahlström A, Felin J, et al. Gut microbiota regulates bile acid metabolism by reducing the levels of tauro-beta-muricholic acid, a naturally occurring FXR antagonist. Cell Metab 2013;17(2):225–35.
58. Björkholm B, Bok CM, Lundin A, et al. Intestinal microbiota regulate xenobiotic metabolism in the liver. PLoS One 2009;4(9):e6958.
59. Gao J, He J, Zhai Y, et al. The constitutive androstane receptor is an anti-obesity nuclear receptor that improves insulin sensitivity. J Biol Chem 2009;284(38): 25984–92.
60. Dong B, Saha PK, Huang W, et al. Activation of nuclear receptor CAR ameliorates diabetes and fatty liver disease. Proc Natl Acad Sci U S A 2009;106(44):18831–6.
61. Moore DD. Physiology: a metabolic minuet. Nature 2013;502(7472):454–5.
62. Kohsaka A, Laposky AD, Ramsey KM, et al. High-fat diet disrupts behavioral and molecular circadian rhythms in mice. Cell Metab 2007;6(5):414–21.
63. Mukherji A, Kobiita A, Ye T, et al. Homeostasis in intestinal epithelium is orchestrated by the circadian clock and microbiota cues transduced by TLRs. Cell 2013;153(4):812–27.
64. Mennigen R, Nolte K, Rijcken E, et al. Probiotic mixture VSL#3 protects the epithelial barrier by maintaining tight junction protein expression and preventing apoptosis in a murine model of colitis. Am J Physiol Gastrointest Liver Physiol 2009;296(5):G1140–9.
65. Wang J, Tang H, Zhang C, et al. Modulation of gut microbiota during probiotic-mediated attenuation of metabolic syndrome in high fat diet-fed mice. ISME J 2015;9(1):1–15.
66. Nilsson A, Johansson E, Ekström L, et al. Effects of a brown beans evening meal on metabolic risk markers and appetite regulating hormones at a subsequent standardized breakfast: a randomized cross-over study. PLoS One 2013;8(4): e59985.
67. Xiao S, Fei N, Pang X, et al. A gut microbiota-targeted dietary intervention for amelioration of chronic inflammation underlying metabolic syndrome. FEMS Microbiol Ecol 2014;87(2):357–67.
68. Ettinger G, MacDonald K, Reid G, et al. The influence of the human microbiome and probiotics on cardiovascular health. Gut Microbes 2014;5(6):719–28.
69. Alisi A, Bedogni G, Baviera G, et al. Randomised clinical trial: the beneficial effects of VSL#3 in obese children with non-alcoholic steatohepatitis. Aliment Pharmacol Ther 2014;39(11):1276–85.
70. Dhiman RK, Rana B, Agrawal S, et al. Probiotic VSL#3 reduces liver disease severity and hospitalization in patients with cirrhosis: a randomized, controlled trial. Gastroenterology 2014;147(6):1327–37.e3.

71. Bakken JS. Fecal bacteriotherapy for recurrent *Clostridium difficile* infection. Anaerobe 2009;15(6):285–9.

72. Tremaroli V, Karlsson F, Werling M, et al. Roux-en-Y gastric bypass and vertical banded gastroplasty induce long-term changes on the human gut microbiome contributing to fat mass regulation. Cell Metab 2015;22(2):228–38.

73. Vrieze A, Van Nood E, Holleman F, et al. Transfer of intestinal microbiota from lean donors increases insulin sensitivity in individuals with metabolic syndrome. Gastroenterology 2012;143(4):913–6.e7.

74. Bakken JS, Borody T, Brandt LJ, et al. Treating *Clostridium difficile* infection with fecal microbiota transplantation. Clin Gastroenterol Hepatol 2011;9(12):1044–9.

75. Tsilingiri K, Barbosa T, Penna G, et al. Probiotic and postbiotic activity in health and disease: comparison on a novel polarised ex-vivo organ culture model. Gut 2012;61(7):1007–15.

Is Obesity Associated with Barrett's Esophagus and Esophageal Adenocarcinoma?

 CrossMark

Kristle Lee Lynch, MD

KEYWORDS

- Barrett's esophagus • Obesity • Central adiposity • Esophageal adenocarcinoma
- Waist-to-hip ratio

KEY POINTS

- Barrett's esophagus is characterized by metaplastic columnar epithelium in the distal esophagus. Esophageal adenocarcinoma can occur from dysplastic progression of Barrett's esophagus.
- There is evidence that Barrett's esophagus is more strongly related to central adiposity and waist-to-hip-ratio than overall obesity.
- Both obesity and the incidence of esophageal adenocarcinoma have increased significantly in the past three decades. Numerous studies have shown an association between obesity and esophageal adenocarcinoma.
- The mechanism by which obesity leads to carcinogenesis involves a complex interplay of inflammatory cytokines and hormones.
- Further studies are warranted to investigate whether weight loss can decrease the risk of Barrett's esophagus and progression to esophageal adenocarcinoma.

INTRODUCTION

The incidence of Barrett's esophagus and esophageal adenocarcinoma (EAC) has increased over the past several decades in the Western world. The rise in obesity paralleled this increase. It is known that obesity predisposes to many different types of malignancy; EAC is one such malignancy.[1,2] Barrett's esophagus is a recent area of investigation given that it is a precursor lesion to EAC. One may assume that Barrett's esophagus shares risk factors with EAC and thus has the same relationship with obesity. However, not all patients with Barrett's esophagus develop esophageal malignancy so its risk factors may be unique.[3] The treatment of Barrett's esophagus is

Disclosure Statement: The author has nothing to disclose.
Division of Gastroenterology and Hepatology, Department of Internal Medicine, The University of Pennsylvania Health System, PCAM 7 South, 3400 Civic Center Boulevard, Philadelphia, PA 19104, USA
E-mail address: Kristle.Lynch@uphs.upenn.edu

Gastroenterol Clin N Am 45 (2016) 615–624
http://dx.doi.org/10.1016/j.gtc.2016.07.002
0889-8553/16/© 2016 Elsevier Inc. All rights reserved.

currently still in evolution and the identification of modifiable risk factors for Barrett's esophagus is crucial in prevention and risk stratification. This article investigates the relationship between obesity and Barrett's esophagus and EAC.

BARRETT'S ESOPHAGUS

Barrett's esophagus is characterized by the replacement of squamous mucosa in the distal esophagus with metaplastic columnar epithelium as a result of chronic exposure of the distal esophagus to acidic gastric contents. Barrett's esophagus can progress to low-grade dysplasia and high-grade dysplasia before ultimately terminating in EAC seen in **Fig. 1**. However, this pathway is not obligatory.[4] Nevertheless, Barrett's esophagus is associated with a 40-fold increase in the risk of EAC over the general population.[5] Thus, the identification of risk factors for Barrett's metaplasia is crucial in attempts to prevent the disease and optimizing treatment selection.

OBESITY AND BARRETT'S ESOPHAGUS

Epidemiologic studies have revealed that the mean body mass index (BMI) is higher in patients with Barrett's esophagus than the general population.[6] Follow-up cross-sectional studies have demonstrated a significant relationship between Barrett's esophagus and obesity.[7] Additionally, it has been shown that increased BMI is associated more strongly with long-segment than short-segment Barrett's esophagus.[6] Therefore, obesity may be a risk factor for Barrett's metaplasia and a possible factor in furthering the progression of metaplasia toward malignancy.

However, recent works suggest that central adiposity may be a more important risk factor for Barrett's esophagus than simply BMI. BMI is clearly not applicable to every patient because it only takes into account weight and height, not necessarily body composition. A population-based study of Washington state residents found that a high waist-to-hip ratio was strongly related to Barrett's esophagus risk (odds ratio [OR], 2.8; 95% confidence interval [CI], 1.5–5.1) but the association between BMI and Barrett's esophagus was not as strong (OR, 1.5; 95% CI, 0.8–2.9). Adjustment for heartburn symptoms did not significantly change this result, suggesting that this relationship may be independent of gastroesophageal reflux disease (GERD).[8]

Abdominal circumference has also been identified as a more precise potential risk factor for Barrett's esophagus. A case control study found a significant association between larger abdominal circumference and Barrett's esophagus (OR, 2.24; 95% CI, 1.21–4.15) and no association with BMI. Factoring in GERD symptoms somewhat attenuated the results, giving an adjusted OR of 1.78 (95% CI, 0.86–3.66).[5] A later case control study revealed similar results; patients with Barrett's esophagus were twice as likely to have a high waist-to-hip ratio as control patients but mean BMI was unrelated. This association between Barrett's esophagus and waist-to-hip ratio was not significantly attenuated when GERD symptoms were factored in.[9]

Finally, a recent meta-analysis found an association between central adiposity and Barrett's esophagus that persisted after adjusting for BMI. This analysis showed that after adjusting for GERD symptoms, patients with central adiposity had double the risk of Barrett's esophagus than those without central adiposity.[10] A summary of the prior studies evaluating central adiposity and obesity in relation to Barrett's esophagus is seen in **Fig. 2**. As displayed, central adiposity indeed seems to be more strongly related to Barrett's esophagus than overall obesity.

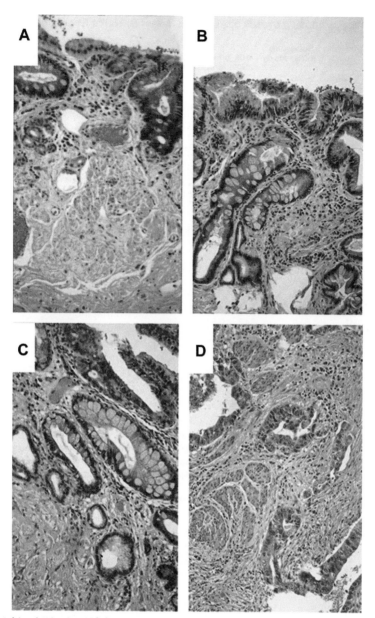

Fig. 1. A histologic view of the Barrett's esophagus progression to esophageal adenocarcinoma (hematoxylin-eosin, original magnification ×100). Barrett's esophagus with no dysplasia (*A*), low-grade dysplasia (*B*), high-grade dysplasia (*C*), and esophageal adenocarcinoma (*D*). (*Courtesy of* Kristen Stashek, MD and Kristle Lynch, MD, Philadelphia, PA.)

OBESITY AND ESOPHAGEAL ADENOCARCINOMA

The incidence of EAC has increased a staggering 600% over the last 30 years.[11] At the same time, the worldwide prevalence of obesity has also increased. **Fig. 3** shows the trends in incidence of EAC and in obesity prevalence. Given the increase in obesity

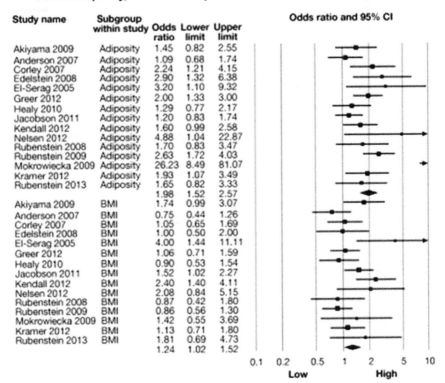

Fig. 2. A summary of the prior studies evaluating the relationship of central adiposity with Barrett's esophagus (*top rows*) and body mass index with Barrett's esophagus (*bottom rows*). (*From* Singh S, Sharma AN, Murad MH, et al. Central adiposity is associated with increased risk of esophageal inflammation, metaplasia, and adenocarcinoma: a systematic review and meta-analysis. Clin Gastroenterol Hepatol 2013;11(11):1407; with permission.)

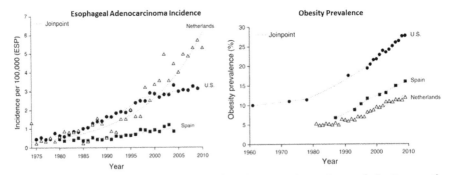

Fig. 3. The trend of incidence of esophageal carcinoma and prevalence of obesity over the past decades. The Netherlands had the most notable increase in incidence of esophageal adenocarcinoma. The United States by far has the highest prevalence of obesity. (*Adapted from* Kroep S, Lansdorp-Vogelaar I, Rubenstein JH, et al. Comparing trends in esophageal adenocarcinoma incidence and lifestyle factors between the United States, Spain, and the Netherlands. Am J Gastroenterol 2014;109(3):338–40; with permission.)

and EAC in the past several decades, numerous studies have examined this relationship. A study based on registry data examined the increase in EAC in the United States, Spain, and the Netherlands. There was a significant increase in all three countries and most significantly in the Netherlands. However, the increase in obesity in these countries over the same time period did not precisely parallel the rise in EAC.[1] Thus it was thought that these trends were not necessarily related.

However, much data to the contrary exist. A meta-analysis and systematic review in 2008 evaluated the relationship of BMI and the risk for 20 different types of cancer. An increase in BMI was associated with EAC. Overall this was the most strongly associated cancer in men and the third most strongly associated cancer in women.[2] To further support this finding, a population-based case control study of more than 1000 patients revealed a clear relationship between BMI and EAC. Patients with a self-reported overweight BMI had a higher risk for EAC than patients with a normal BMI; this risk increased as the BMI increased. Impressively, obese patients with a BMI greater than 40 had a six-fold increase in their risk of EAC over patients with a normal BMI.[12] Likewise, a meta-analysis and a prospective survey study of almost 500,000 patients found that a BMI greater than 30 was associated with double the risk of EAC.[13,14]

As evidenced by these large-scale studies that have similar results, there is a clear link between obesity and EAC. There have been only a few studies specifically investigating central adiposity in EAC. An international population-based study found that EAC was related to a larger waist circumference but not BMI.[15] However, two contrasting studies revealed that general obesity and a larger waist circumference were associated with an increase in EAC.[16,17] Thus, it is not clear that central obesity is a more precise risk factor for EAC than general obesity and this may be an area for future studies.

MECHANISM OF CARCINOGENESIS

A logical mechanism for the relationship between obesity, Barrett's esophagus, and EAC is the pathway of GERD. Obesity causes increased intra-abdominal pressure and an increased risk of hiatal hernia. When pressure and distention in the stomach increase, transient lower esophageal sphincter relaxations are triggered; this facilities the retrograde movement of gastric contents into the distal esophagus. As seen in **Fig. 4**, increased intragastric pressure and decreased intraesophageal pressure can cause an elevated gastroesophageal pressure gradient. Chronic reflux can predispose to Barrett's esophagus, which may progress via the dysplasia pathway to EAC.[11] However, adjusting the odds ratios for GERD does not typically result in diminished effects. Thus there is evidence that the relationship between obesity and Barrett's esophagus and EAC may be independent of GERD.

There are multiple pathways by which obesity can lead to cell turnover and tumor growth. Increased adipose tissue has been shown to increase systemic levels of inflammatory cytokines, such as leptin.[18] Adipose tissue has also been shown to release free fatty acids, tumor necrosis factor-α, and resistin; this leads to the development of insulin resistance. Chronically elevated insulin and insulin-like growth factor levels can promote cellular proliferation while inhibiting apoptosis, providing a possible mechanism for carcinogenesis.[19] Adiponectin is typically decreased in central and overall obesity and insulin resistant states. Adiponectin induces apoptosis, inhibits cell-cycle progression, and inhibits growth factors.[20] Thus in obesity, a decrease in adiponectin can contribute to carcinogenesis via decreased inhibition of proliferation. These mechanisms are outlined in **Fig. 5**.

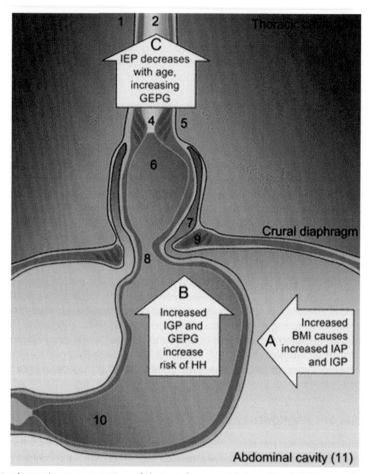

Fig. 4. A schematic representation of the esophagogastric junction (EGJ) in a patient with a hiatal hernia (HH) demonstrating how an elevated intra-abdominal pressure (IAP) in patients with high BMI (*arrow A*) increases intragastric pressure (IGP) (*arrow B*). The numbers denote the various structures, compartments, and pressures influencing the transit of gastric contents across the EGJ. 1, esophageal body: length, contractility, and motility patterns; 2, intraesophageal pressure (IEP); 3, intrathoracic pressure; 4, EGJ diameter; 5, lower esophageal sphincter: basal pressure and transient relaxations; 6, pressure in hiatal sac; 7, pressure in herniated peritoneal sac; 8, length of herniated portion of stomach; 9, crural diaphragm: muscle tone and hiatal diameter; 10, IGP; 11, intra-abdominal pressure. GEPG, gastroesophageal pressure gradients. (*From* de Vries DR, van Herwaarden MA, Smout AJ, et al. Gastroesophageal pressure gradients in gastroesophageal reflux disease: relations with hiatal hernia, body mass index, and esophageal acid exposure. Am J Gastroenterol 2008;103(6):1353; with permission.)

To date, these mechanisms have not been proven. A recent study compared leptin and ghrelin levels of patients with Barrett's esophagus with a matched control group. Increases in ghrelin were associated with an increased risk of Barrett's esophagus, whereas leptin was inversely associated with this risk.[21] However, the Seattle Barrett's esophagus study found that increased leptin levels were associated with increased progression to EAC.[22] Thus the interplay of hormones may not be straightforward and further studies are warranted to elucidate this relationship.

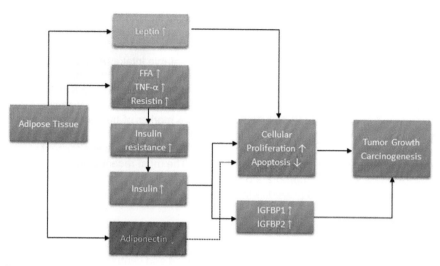

Fig. 5. Possible mechanisms by which an increase in adipose tissue can lead to insulin resistance and eventual tumor growth. FFA, free fatty acid; TNF, tumor necrosis factor.

Additionally, if obesity is a risk factor for Barrett's esophagus and EAC it is possible that weight loss could contribute to regression of disease. Currently, strong data to illustrate this point do not exist. However, a series of five patients with long-segment Barrett's esophagus who underwent Roux-en-y gastric bypass noted a drop in mean BMI from 43 to 33 and an improvement in their metaplasia. Specifically, two patients had low-grade dysplasia and one patient was indeterminate for dysplasia before their surgery. At their 1-year postoperative upper endoscopy, only one patient had dysplasia and the length of Barrett's mucosa decreased in four of the five patients.[23] Although this was an isolated and small-scale study, the results were favorable. Given the relationship with obesity as described previously and the increased incidence of Barrett's esophagus over the past decades, larger prospective studies evaluating the role of weight loss in the progression of Barrett's esophagus are warranted.

DIETARY IMPACT

There have been many studies on the role of diet in Barrett's esophagus and EAC. Dietary nitrites have been identified and publicized as a potential risk factor for many types of malignancy.[24] They are found naturally in high quantities in green leafy vegetables and are often added to processed meats. Nitrites are converted into nitrous oxide in the presence of gastric acid, and in the epithelium of esophagus can lead to the production of N-nitroso products, which are potential carcinogens. However, most dietary nitrite is absorbed by the small bowel and eventually excreted as urine.[25] To date, several studies examining this relationship have not found a significant association between nitrite intake and EAC.[26]

More specifically, there have been studies evaluating nitrate-containing meat consumption and EAC. A study by Rogers and colleagues[24] revealed a slightly increased odds ratio of 1.82 in patients with high nitrate-containing meat intake. However, a more recent publication out of the Netherlands found no relationship between meat consumption or nitrite consumption with Barrett's esophagus.[27] Thus if the risk of

EAC is indeed increased by diets high in nitrite-containing meats, it is not likely mediated via the Barrett's esophagus pathway; further studies are needed to clarify this relationship.

Another dietary factor of interest is fruit and vegetable intake. A population-based case-control study reported the attributable risk of low fruit and vegetable intake to EAC to be 15.3%.[28] However, a prospective survey study by George and colleagues[29] found no association between fruit and vegetable intake and EAC. It was suggested that fruit and vegetable intake may be a surrogate marker of health consciousness, smoking, or other potential confounding factors.

Although a diet tailored to prevent Barrett's esophagus and the development of EAC would be ideal, it is unfortunately far from reality. The most recent guidelines for Barrett's esophagus do not incorporate diet into risk factors or recommend specific dietary strategies for disease prevention.[30]

SUMMARY

Barrett's esophagus, EAC, and obesity have all increased dramatically over the past several decades. Based on current data, generalized and central obesity are risk factors for Barrett's esophagus and general obesity is a risk factor for EAC. BMI is not applicable to every patient and abdominal obesity specifically may play a more important role. Given that men have a higher prevalence of central obesity than women; this finding may account for the gender disproportionate incidence of Barrett's esophagus and possibly EAC. Adipose tissue leads to an increase in cellular proliferation and decrease in apoptosis via multiple mechanisms. Further studies are warranted to prove these mechanisms and clarify markers to assist in risk stratification and treatment timing in the future. There are no current preventative dietary guidelines for these diseases. Weight loss is a great potential target for disease prevention but studies have not yet proven this to be effective.

REFERENCES

1. Kroep S, Lansdorp-Vogelaar I, Rubenstein JH, et al. Comparing trends in esophageal adenocarcinoma incidence and lifestyle factors between the United States, Spain, and the Netherlands. Am J Gastroenterol 2014;109(3):336–43.
2. Renehan AG, Tyson M, Egger M, et al. Body-mass index and incidence of cancer: a systematic review and meta-analysis of prospective observational studies. Lancet 2008;371(9612):569–78.
3. Lada MJ, Nieman DR, Han M, et al. Gastroesophageal reflux disease, proton-pump inhibitor use and Barrett's esophagus in esophageal adenocarcinoma: trends revisited. Surgery 2013;154(4):856–64.
4. Falk GW. Barrett's oesophagus: frequency and prediction of dysplasia and cancer. Best Pract Res Clin Gastroenterol 2015;29(1):125–38.
5. Corley DA, Kubo A, Levin TR, et al. Abdominal obesity and body mass index as risk factors for Barrett's esophagus. Gastroenterology 2007;133(1):34–41.
6. Abdallah J, Maradey-Romero C, Lewis S, et al. The relationship between length of Barrett's oesophagus mucosa and body mass index. Aliment Pharmacol Ther 2015;41(1):137–44.
7. Stein DJ, El-Serag HB, Kuczynski J, et al. The association of body mass index with Barrett's oesophagus. Aliment Pharmacol Ther 2005;22(10):1005–10.
8. Edelstein ZR, Farrow DC, Bronner MP, et al. Central adiposity and risk of Barrett's esophagus. Gastroenterology 2007;133(2):403–11.

9. Kramer JR, Fischbach LA, Richardson P, et al. Waist-to-hip ratio, but not body mass index, is associated with an increased risk of Barrett's esophagus in white men. Clin Gastroenterol Hepatol 2013;11(4):373–81.e1.

10. Singh S, Sharma AN, Murad MH, et al. Central adiposity is associated with increased risk of esophageal inflammation, metaplasia, and adenocarcinoma: a systematic review and meta-analysis. Clin Gastroenterol Hepatol 2013;11(11): 1399–412.

11. Alexandre L, Long E, Beales IL. Pathophysiological mechanisms linking obesity and esophageal adenocarcinoma. World J Gastrointest Pathophysiol 2014;5(4): 534–49.

12. Whiteman DC, Sadeghi S, Pandeya N, et al, Australian Cancer Study. Combined effects of obesity, acid reflux and smoking on the risk of adenocarcinomas of the esophagus. Gut 2008;57(2):173–80.

13. Kubo A, Corley DA. Body mass index and adenocarcinomas of the esophagus or gastric cardia: a systematic review and meta-analysis. Cancer Epidemiol Biomarkers Prev 2006;15(5):872–8.

14. Abnet CC, Freedman ND, Hollenbeck AR, et al. A prospective study of BMI and risk of oesophageal and gastric adenocarcinoma. Eur J Cancer 2008;44(3): 465–71.

15. Steffen A, Huerta JM, Weiderpass E, et al. General and abdominal obesity and risk of esophageal and gastric adenocarcinoma in the European prospective investigation into cancer and nutrition. Int J Cancer 2015;137(3):646–57.

16. MacInnis RJ, English DR, Hopper JL, et al. Body size and composition and the risk of gastric and oesophageal adenocarcinoma. Int J Cancer 2006;118(10): 2628–31.

17. Corley DA, Kubo A, Zhao W. Abdominal obesity and the risk of esophageal and gastric cardia carcinomas. Cancer Epidemiol Biomarkers Prev 2008;17(2):352–8.

18. Drahos J, Ricker W, Parsons R, et al. Metabolic syndrome increases risk of Barrett esophagus in the absence of gastroesophageal reflux: an analysis of SEER-Medicare data. J Clin Gastroenterol 2015;49(4):282–8.

19. Calle EE, Kaaks R. Overweight, obesity and cancer: epidemiological evidence and proposed mechanisms. Nat Rev Cancer 2004;4(8):579–91.

20. Murray L, Romero Y. Role of obesity in Barrett's esophagus and cancer. Surg Oncol Clin N Am 2009;18(3):439–52.

21. Thomas SJ, Almers L, Schneider J, et al. Ghrelin and leptin have a complex relationship with risk of Barrett's esophagus. Dig Dis Sci 2016;61(1):70–9.

22. Duggan C, Onstad L, Hardikar S, et al. Association between markers of obesity and progression from Barrett's esophagus to esophageal adenocarcinoma. Clin Gastroenterol Hepatol 2013;11:934–43.

23. Houghton SG, Romero Y, Sarr MG. Effect of roux-en-y gastric bypass in obese patients with Barrett's esophagus: attempts to eliminate duodenogastric reflux. Surg Obes Relat Dis 2008;4(1):1–4 [discussion: 4–5].

24. Rogers MA, Vaughan TL, Davis S, et al. Consumption of nitrate, nitrite, and nitrosodimethylamine and the risk of upper aerodigestive tract cancer. Cancer Epidemiol Biomarkers Prev 1995;4(1):29–36.

25. Iijima K, Grant J, McElroy K, et al. Novel mechanism of nitrosative stress from dietary nitrate with relevance to gastro-oesophageal junction cancers. Carcinogenesis 2003;24(12):1951–60.

26. Keszei AP, Goldbohm RA, Schouten LJ, et al. Dietary N-nitroso compounds, endogenous nitrosation, and the risk of esophageal and gastric cancer subtypes in the Netherlands cohort study. Am J Clin Nutr 2013;97(1):135–46.

27. Keszei AP, Schouten LJ, Driessen AL, et al. Meat consumption and the risk of Barrett's esophagus in a large Dutch cohort. Cancer Epidemiol Biomarkers Prev 2013;22(6):1162–6.
28. Engel LS, Chow WH, Vaughan TL, et al. Population attributable risks of esophageal and gastric cancers. J Natl Cancer Inst 2003;95(18):1404–13.
29. George SM, Park Y, Leitzmann MF, et al. Fruit and vegetable intake and risk of cancer: a prospective cohort study. Am J Clin Nutr 2009;89(1):347–53.
30. Shaheen NJ, Falk GW, Iyer PG, et al, American College of Gastroenterology. ACG clinical guideline: diagnosis and management of Barrett's esophagus. Am J Gastroenterol 2016;111(1):30–50 [quiz: 51].

The Impact of Obesity on Gallstone Disease, Acute Pancreatitis, and Pancreatic Cancer

Zobeida Cruz-Monserrate, PhD[a,b], Darwin L. Conwell, MD, MS[a], Somashekar G. Krishna, MD, MPH[a],*

KEYWORDS

• Obesity • Gallstone disease • Pancreatitis • Pancreatic cancer

KEY POINTS

• Obesity is frequently associated with gallstone disease, acute pancreatitis, liver steatosis, and gastrointestinal cancers.
• The formation of gallstones in patients with obesity is multifactorial. A rapid weight loss in obesity also predisposes patients to gallstone formation.
• Obese patients are at increased risk of severe acute pancreatitis. Multiple local and systemic factors contribute to poor outcomes in patients with obesity.
• Although recognized as a risk factor for pancreatic cancer, obesity is also associated with poor outcomes after surgery for pancreatic cancer.

INTRODUCTION

Obesity is increasing worldwide and the World Health Organization has confirmed this as a global epidemic.[1] Approximately 30% of the world's population is overweight or obese, and no country has reduced its obesity rates in 33 years.[2] In the United States, approximately 78.6 million (34.9%) of adults are obese, a statistic that has doubled over the past 2 decades.[3] In particular, the prevalence of morbid obesity has rapidly increased with an approximate 70% increment from 2000 to 2010.[4] Furthermore,

Grant Support: This publication was supported (D.L. Conwell) by the National Institutes of Diabetes and Digestive and Kidney Diseases and National Cancer Institute under Award Number U01DK108327.
Disclosures: There are no relevant conflicts of interest to report for any author.
^a Section of Pancreatic Diseases, Division of Gastroenterology, Hepatology and Nutrition, The Ohio State University Wexner Medical Center, 395 West 12th Avenue, 2nd Floor, Columbus, OH, USA; ^b The James Comprehensive Cancer Center, The Ohio State University Wexner Medical Center, Columbus, OH, USA
* Corresponding author.
E-mail address: somashekar.krishna@osumc.edu

childhood obesity has more than doubled in children and quadrupled in adolescents in the past 3 decades and this has led to increases in disease rates associated with obesity.[3]

Other than contributing to the metabolic syndrome and cardiorespiratory comorbidities, obesity is frequently associated with gallstone disease, acute pancreatitis, liver steatosis, and gastrointestinal cancers.[5–7] Gallstone disease is highly prevalent (10%–15% of population) in the Western population and is increasing. In the United States, there were 389,180 hospitalizations in 2012 due to cholelithiasis with cholecystitis.[8,9] Acute pancreatitis is the most common single gastrointestinal diagnosis for inpatient hospitalization (275,170 hospitalizations in 2012) and costs an estimated 2.6 billion dollars per year in inpatient costs.[10] The prevalence of inpatient hospitalization for acute pancreatitis is increasing annually, which parallels the rising prevalence of obesity.[4,11] There is an established association between obesity and the development of complications in acute pancreatitis.[12,13] In addition, obesity increases the risk of developing pancreas cancer in particular, pancreatic ductal adenocarcinoma (PDAC).[14–16] PDAC is a devastating disease, with a dismal long-term survival.[17,18] Surgery offers the only possibility of approximating a cure; however, only 20% of patients are eligible because the cancer tends to be detected at a late stage and has already metastasized at diagnosis. In 2016, PDAC became the third leading cause of cancer-related death in the United States and it is projected to become the second by 2030, due to both an aging population and the obesity epidemic.[2,17,19,20]

The aim of this review is to describe the pathophysiology and outcomes of obesity and the association with gallstone disease, acute pancreatitis, and pancreatic cancer.

CHOLELITHIASIS AND OBESITY

There are multiple risk factors for gallstones in patients with obesity (**Table 1**). Although elevated body mass index (BMI) is associated with gallstone disease, a causal association has been demonstrated between increasing BMI and symptomatic gallstones using a mendelian randomization approach.[21] Furthermore, increasing BMI was associated with a 3-fold increment in the risk of cholelithiasis as evidenced in the Nurses' Health Study involving women between 30 and 55 years of age followed over a total of 18 years.[22] A 2.5-fold increase in risk has also been demonstrated among men between 40 and 55 years of age.[23] As an outcome of obesity-associated gallstone disease, the risk of gallbladder cancer also increases with BMI.[24] The lithogenic mechanisms of obesity are multifold and are depicted in **Fig. 1**. These mechanisms can either act alone or contribute in combination. It is of relevance that the presence of components of metabolic syndrome increases the risk of gallstones; a risk of 5% without the presence of metabolic syndrome increases to 25% when all the components are present in a patient.[25]

CHOLELITHIASIS AFTER WEIGHT LOSS IN OBESITY

The trend of bariatric surgeries and simultaneous cholecystectomies in the United States (2005–2011) is shown in **Fig. 2**. Concomitant cholecystectomy during gastric bypass surgery is no longer the routine practice because the operative time, postoperative hospital stay, and postoperative morbidity and mortality are higher with prophylactic cholecystectomy.[26] Several studies have indicated its use only in cases of symptomatic gallbladder disease, in particular cholelithiasis.[27] Concomitant

Table 1
Risk factors and pathophysiology of gallstones in obesity

Disease or Condition	Pathophysiology	Type of Gallstone
Pregnancy Oral contraceptives Estrogen therapy	• Gallbladder stasis • Supersaturated bile	Cholesterol
Total parental nutrition Octreotide administration Calcineurin inhibitors Fibrates	• Inhibition of cholecystokinin • Gallbladder stasis • Supersaturated bile • Inhibition of hepatic bile salt pump • Bile concentration	Cholesterol
Liver cirrhosis	• Hyperestrogenism • Gallbladder stasis • Bile salt malabsorption • Increased enterohepatic circulation of bilirubin	Cholesterol/black pigment
Crohn disease Extended ileal resection Cystic fibrosis	• Increased biliary concentration • Increased enterohepatic circulation of bilirubin	Cholesterol/black pigment
Hemolytic anemia Sickle cell anemia	• Increased calcium bilirubinate • Gallbladder stasis	Black pigment
Alcohol excess	• Reduced bile acid synthesis	Black pigment
Specific ethnic groups (Pima Indians): obesity with diabetes mellitus	• Genetic predisposition	Cholesterol

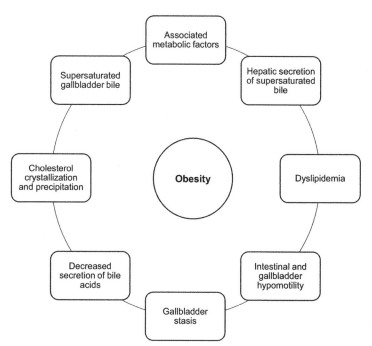

Fig. 1. Pathogenesis of gallstones in obesity: multifactorial mechanisms that could contribute to lithogenesis.

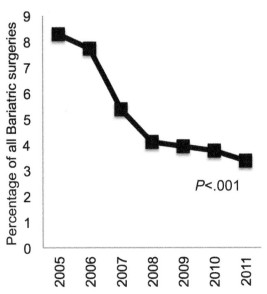

Fig. 2. Trends in types of bariatric surgeries and frequency of concomitant cholecystectomies.

cholecystectomy (2005–2011) has significantly decreased from 8.3% (9880 of 119,382) to 3.4% (3653 of 108,354) for all types of bariatric surgeries (P<.001).[28] After bariatric surgery, the incidence of gallstones or sludge is higher compared with the overall population, ranging from 28% to 71%.[29,30]

PATHOGENESIS OF OBESITY-ASSOCIATED CHOLELITHIASIS

Multiple factors (see **Fig. 1**) may contribute to the increased risk of cholesterol gallstones in obese persons. Because the estimated amount of cholesterol synthesized in the liver is related to body fat, there is increased hepatic secretion of cholesterol in obesity.[31] After this, the bile is saturated with excess cholesterol.[32] Frequently, obese patients have impaired gallbladder motility, which is evident at an early stage of gallstone formation.[33] Due to a combination of these factors, there is aggregation of solid cholesterol crystals and eventual stone formation. This entire process is accelerated in obese patients with weight loss. Other contributing mechanisms include enhanced mobilization of cholesterol, reduced hepatic secretion of biliary bile salts due to decreased hepatic bile acid pool, reduced gallbladder contractility, and increased secretion of biliary calcium.[34,35]

MANAGEMENT OF CHOLELITHIASIS

The management of cholelithiasis in obesity is similar to that in the general population. The classic symptoms of upper abdominal pain, which is acute, and characteristic of a biliary colic prompt further investigations. Liver enzymes and an abdominal ultrasound are initial investigations. In the presence of bile duct dilation and/or liver enzyme abnormality, magnetic resonance cholangiopancreatography (MRCP) should be considered if ultrasound has not detected common bile duct stones. If MRCP does not facilitate an accurate diagnosis, then endoscopic ultrasound should be considered.[36] Asymptomatic gallstones with a normal gallbladder and unremarkable-appearing biliary tree do not need further treatment unless patients develop symptoms. Patients with symptomatic gallstones, however, should be offered cholecystectomy and both asymptomatic choledocholithiasis and symptomatic choledocholithiasis require bile duct clearance prior to cholecystectomy.[36]

Although laparoscopic cholecystectomy is the recommended procedure, it is sometimes not possible in morbidly obese patients. The abdominal wall thickness might prohibit maneuverability of trocars requiring longer devices, additional trocars, and procedural modifications to avoid trocar displacement, abdominal wall insufflation, and subcutaneous emphysema.[37] If surgery is prohibitive due to associated comorbidities, oral litholysis with hydrophilic ursodeoxycholic acid (UDCA) can be considered in patients with small (<5 mm), radiolucent gallstones in patients with a patent cystic duct, although there is a higher rate of recurrence of gallstones.[5,38] Although a majority of weight loss surgeries involve Roux-en-Y gastric bypass (RYGB), the incidence of sleeve gastrectomy has increased in the past 5 years. Despite lower weight loss in sleeve gastrectomy, it has been demonstrated that the incidence of cholecystectomy was similar for both groups of patients at 2-year follow-up after surgery.[39] Rapid weight loss after aggressive diet regimens and gastric by-pass surgery warrants prophylaxis to prevent gallstone formation. The benefit of prophylaxis with oral UDCA has been demonstrated in multiple randomized clinical trials.[40]

ACUTE PANCREATITIS AND OBESITY

Prior population-based studies have demonstrated that the incidence of acute pancreatitis in the United States has been increasing.[41,42] This is true for both emergency department visits and hospital admissions.[41] Despite the increase in incidence, the mortality rate is reportedly lower in the past decade (1% vs 3%–5%).[11,41–43] A majority of patients with acute pancreatitis resolve without associated complications. Approximately 20% of patients with acute pancreatitis, however, are severe, with associated local and systemic complications, including pancreatic walled-off necrosis, compartment syndrome, development of acute kidney injury, and acute respiratory distress syndrome.[44] Presence of persistent organ failure constitutes severe acute pancreatitis, which is associated with a higher mortality of approximately 30%.[44]

Several epidemiologic studies suggest obesity or increased intra-abdominal fat is associated with severe acute pancreatitis and morbid obesity is associated with increased in-hospital mortality in acute pancreatitis.[6,45,46] Previous single-center studies have revealed correlations between increasing BMI and disease severity, including organ dysfunction, infection, pancreatic necrosis, length of hospital stay, and use of intensive care.[47–53] Four meta-analyses published within the past 10 years demonstrate that morbid obesity is independently associated with mortality in acute pancreatitis.[47,48,54,55] Most recently, a large Japanese population-based inpatient study demonstrated independent risk of mortality in class 2 and 3 obesity.[56]

PATHOGENESIS OF ACUTE PANCREATITIS IN OBESITY

Obese patients are at increased risk of severe acute pancreatitis.[49] Multiple local and systemic factors have been implicated in the pathogenesis of adverse prognostication in obesity (**Fig. 3**). There is evidence of increased pancreatic fat in patients with increasing BMI.[57–59] It has also been shown that pancreatic fat has a direct toxic effect on the parenchyma of the pancreas.[58,59] New evidence indicates that fat composition

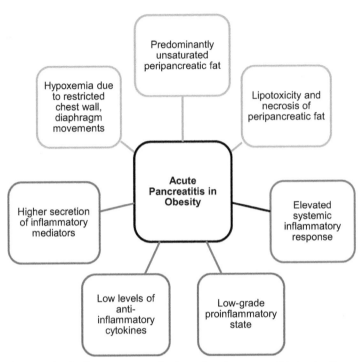

Fig. 3. Pathogenesis of adverse prognostication of acute pancreatitis in obesity: multifactorial mechanisms involving local (*green box*) and systemic (*blue box*) factors.

in obesity is predominantly unsaturated and that lipolysis worsens local and systemic injury. The cytokine increase in severe acute pancreatitis is thought to be secondary to lipotoxicity.[60] It has also been demonstrated that deposits of intra-abdominal peripancreatic fat in obese patients undergo necrosis during acute pancreatitis and this contributes to the spectrum of necrotizing pancreatitis.[61] Furthermore, a recent publication demonstrated that peripancreatic fat lipolysis resulted in multisystem injury independent of pancreatic necrosis.[62] Obesity in itself constitutes a low-grade proinflammatory state. A higher level of proinflammatory cytokines, such as tumor necrosis factor (TNF)-α, interleukin (IL)-10, IL-6, IL-1β, and plasminogen activator inhibitor-1 have been described.[12,13] Hence, the inflammatory response is increased and there is an up-regulation of the proinflammatory cytokines that leads to a larger inflammatory response.

In addition to the role of pancreatic and peripancreatic necrosis and inflammatory hypothesis, there is a restriction of chest wall and diaphragmatic movements that leads to decrease in inspiratory capacity and has the net effect of increasing physiologic pulmonary arteriovenous shunting, thus leading to hypoxemia. In acute pancreatitis, hypoxemia produces an oxygen deficit and exacerbates the underlying cellular damage from the inflammatory response, which subsequently increases the rate of multiorgan failure and death.[47]

ACUTE PANCREATITIS AND WEIGHT LOSS IN OBESITY

Bariatric surgery in acute pancreatitis is not adversely associated with in-hospital mortality or development of organ failure and thus may mitigate the obesity-associated adverse prognostication in acute pancreatitis.[28] Several studies, including a recent meta-analysis, have shown a decrease in IL-6, C-reactive protein, and TNF-α after bariatric surgery.[63,64] The decrease in proinflammatory biomarkers and increase in anti-inflammatory mediators have been shown independent of the extent of weight loss.[65] Thus, it is biologically plausible that weight loss in obesity could contribute to a decrease in mortality and improved clinical outcomes when such patients develop acute pancreatitis. In a recent analysis of a large population, patients with prior bariatric surgery incurred fewer incidents of respiratory failure and mechanical ventilation. A potential explanation is improved inspiratory capacity by lesser restriction of diaphragmatic and chest wall movements, thus preventing hypoxemia and related inflammation-induced cellular damage.[47] Further exploration of these interesting findings in a prospective cohort might provide additional insights into the mechanisms of obesity and related weight loss in the pathogenesis and management of acute pancreatitis.

GALLSTONE DISEASE AND ACUTE PANCREATITIS IN OBESITY AND IMPACT OF WEIGHT LOSS SURGERY

Although gallstones are one of the most common causes of acute pancreatitis, only 3.4% of patients in a large cohort of a general population developed acute pancreatitis over a 20-year period.[66] After weight-loss surgery, the incidence of gallstones or sludge is higher compared with the overall population, ranging from 28% to 71%.[29,30] The prevalence of biliary pancreatitis in a recent meta-analysis of 13 studies involving RYGB surgery (without concomitant cholecystectomy) was 0.2%.[26] Results from prior studies including a recent population-based analysis show that 0.25% of all patients with prior RYGB are diagnosed with gallstone-associated acute pancreatitis.[26,28] These rates were however higher (1.04%) in a recent publication from a single tertiary care center, but most cases were mild with favorable outcomes.[67] Despite these findings, there is continuing declining trend in concomitant cholecystectomy and the authors do not expect any changes in these trends because acute pancreatitis has better outcomes after weight loss surgery.

OBESITY AND PANCREATIC CANCER RISK

Obesity is a significant risk factor for pancreatic cancer, in particular, PDAC.[68–72] This is concerning, because obesity rates are increasing worldwide, mostly due to increased consumption of a Western-style diet, high in fat and calories.[2] A projection of the future health and economic burden of obesity in 2030 estimated that continuation of existing increasing trends in obesity will lead to approximately 500,000 additional cases of cancer in the United States by 2030.[7] Obesity not only increases cancer risk but also may reduce survival of cancer patients.[18] Epidemiologic data indicates that premorbid obesity (at least 1 year before diagnosis of pancreatic cancer) adversely influences PDAC-related mortality in a dose-dependent manner.[18] In addition, a high BMI has been associated with the risk of PDAC, age at onset, and overall survival.[18] Most studies have positively associated BMI with pancreatic cancer incidence and mortality.[70,73–76] A meta-analysis and a pooled analysis with pancreatic cancer cases reported a 10% and 14% increase in risk for each 5 kg/m^2 incremental increase in BMI, respectively.[77,78] A more recent study observed positive associations among measures of central obesity, waist circumference, and waist-to-hip ratio with pancreatic cancer mortality.[79] Currently, BMI does not influence treatment options for patients with PDAC because these options are already limited for these patients. Moreover, little is known about the effects of weight loss in decreasing risk of PDAC development or improving prognosis.

OBESITY AND PANCREATIC SURGERY OUTCOMES

Because most patients with PDAC are first diagnosed when the disease has already spread, only 20% of patients are detected at a stage were surgical resection is an option. Surgery for PDAC may be combined with other types of treatment, such as radiation therapy and/or chemotherapy. Pancreatic surgical resection is a complex surgery for which mortality rates has widely decreased over the years.[80] Complications rates after pancreatic resections, however, remain high and several studies have related an elevated BMI to a higher risk of overall surgical complications and onset of pancreatic fistula.[81,82] A recent study determined that increase adipose tissue in particular visceral adiposity is a determinant of postoperative morbidity.[83] Moreover, other studies showed that sarcopenic obesity and myosteatosis were correlated with worse long-term survival.[70] In addition, a combination of visceral obesity and sarcopenia was also shown a good predictor of death postsurgery, whereas visceral fat area was an independent predictor of pancreatic fistula.[73] In patients with advance PDAC, the presence of sarcopenia in overweight and obese patients was an independent indicator of adverse prognosis and it was suggested that it needs to be considered in the stratification of patients that participate in clinical trials.[74]

OBESITY-INDUCED PANCREATIC CANCER MECHANISMS

Most of the current mechanistic studies on obesity and PDAC development have been performed in a preclinical setting, using genetically engineered mouse models (GEMMs) that mimic the progression of the human disease. These models have helped identify novel mechanisms that otherwise are difficult to discover in human trials, due to their long-term duration. In some of these studies using GEMMs, it has been shown that diet-induced obesity acts as an inflammatory stimulus to trigger increased Kirsten rat sarcoma viral oncogene homolog (KRas) activity.[84] Cyclooxygenase 2 was also found critical in the inflammatory loop that leads to inflammation, increased fibrotic stroma, activation of KRas downstream signaling pathways, increased development of pancreatic intraepithelial neoplasia lesions, and decreased mice survival.[84] Treatment with a cyclooxygenase 2 inhibitor (celecoxib) decreased the effects observed in these animals after diet-induced obesity.[84] This study was in agreement with other groups that looked at the effects of diet-induced obesity in various GEMM models using different sources and concentrations of fats in accelerating PDAC development.[85–87]

OBESITY AND PANCREAS CANCER: GAPS AND FUTURE RESEARCH

Although there have been many epidemiologic studies indicating the dangers of obesity in promoting PDAC and affecting surgical outcomes, many basic questions about the mechanisms of how this occurs remain unanswered. Therefore, now more than ever, a better understanding is needed of the molecular mechanisms that link obesity and PDAC development. Further insight into this relationship will allow developing and integrating novel preventative approaches focused on modifiable risk factors. Recently, it was suggested that there may be a large window of opportunity (approximately 11 years) for the detection of PDAC while the disease is in its earliest and most treatable stages.[17,88] This suggests that an opportunity exists for improving outcomes via adopting preventative approaches in a subset of patients, especially obese individuals.

SUMMARY

If the current trend of obesity continues, it would lead to persistent adverse prognostication of acute pancreatitis and an increased prevalence of gallstone disease and pancreatic adenocarcinoma. Most recent literature suggests increasing prevalence of obesity in children and adolescents; thus, in the near future, a younger patient population with cholesterol cholelithiasis and pancreatic disease, including adenocarcinoma, may be treated. Current and future research should focus on increasing and improving operative, endoscopic, and noninvasive interventions for effectively restricting the uncontrolled global increase in prevalence of obesity.

REFERENCES

1. Obesity: preventing and managing the global epidemic. Report of a WHO consultation. World Health Organ Tech Rep Ser 2000;894:i–xii, 1–253.
2. Ng M, Fleming T, Robinson M, et al. Global, regional, and national prevalence of overweight and obesity in children and adults during 1980-2013: a systematic analysis for the Global Burden of Disease Study 2013. Lancet 2014;384:766–81.
3. Ogden CL, Carroll MD, Kit BK, et al. Prevalence of childhood and adult obesity in the United States, 2011-2012. JAMA 2014;311:806–14.
4. Sturm R, Hattori A. Morbid obesity rates continue to rise rapidly in the United States. Int J Obes (Lond) 2013;37:889–91.
5. Portincasa P, Moschetta A, Palasciano G. Cholesterol gallstone disease. Lancet 2006;368:230–9.
6. Krishna SG, Hinton A, Oza V, et al. Morbid obesity is associated with adverse clinical outcomes in acute pancreatitis: a propensity-matched study. Am J Gastroenterol 2015;110:1608–19.
7. Wang YC, McPherson K, Marsh T, et al. Health and economic burden of the projected obesity trends in the USA and the UK. Lancet 2011;378:815–25.
8. Stinton LM, Myers RP, Shaffer EA. Epidemiology of gallstones. Gastroenterol Clin North Am 2010;39:157–69, vii.
9. Peery AF, Crockett SD, Barritt AS, et al. Burden of gastrointestinal, liver, and pancreatic diseases in the United States. Gastroenterology 2015;149: 1731–1741 e3.
10. Peery AF, Dellon ES, Lund J, et al. Burden of gastrointestinal disease in the United States: 2012 update. Gastroenterology 2012;143:1179–1187 e1–3.
11. Fagenholz PJ, Castillo CF, Harris NS, et al. Increasing United States hospital admissions for acute pancreatitis, 1988-2003. Ann Epidemiol 2007;17:491–7.
12. Fain JN, Madan AK, Hiler ML, et al. Comparison of the release of adipokines by adipose tissue, adipose tissue matrix, and adipocytes from visceral and subcutaneous abdominal adipose tissues of obese humans. Endocrinology 2004;145: 2273–82.
13. Lee YH, Pratley RE. The evolving role of inflammation in obesity and the metabolic syndrome. Curr Diab Rep 2005;5:70–5.
14. Renehan AG, Zwahlen M, Egger M. Adiposity and cancer risk: new mechanistic insights from epidemiology. Nat Rev Cancer 2015;15:484–98.
15. Allott EH, Hursting SD. Obesity and cancer: mechanistic insights from transdisciplinary studies. Endocr Relat Cancer 2015;22:R365–86.
16. Font-Burgada J, Sun B, Karin M. Obesity and cancer: the oil that feeds the flame. Cell Metab 2016;23:48–62.
17. Siegel RL, Miller KD, Jemal A. Cancer statistics, 2016. CA Cancer J Clin 2016; 66:7–30.

18. Majumder K, Gupta A, Arora N, et al. Premorbid obesity and mortality in patients with pancreatic cancer: a systematic review and meta-analysis. Clin Gastroenterol Hepatol 2016;14:355–368.e.

19. Smith BD, Smith GL, Hurria A, et al. Future of cancer incidence in the United States: burdens upon an aging, changing nation. J Clin Oncol 2009;27:2758–65.

20. Rahib L, Smith BD, Aizenberg R, et al. Projecting cancer incidence and deaths to 2030: the unexpected burden of thyroid, liver, and pancreas cancers in the United States. Cancer Res 2014;74:2913–21.

21. Stender S, Nordestgaard BG, Tybjaerg-Hansen A. Elevated body mass index as a causal risk factor for symptomatic gallstone disease: a Mendelian randomization study. Hepatology 2013;58:2133–41.

22. Stampfer MJ, Maclure KM, Colditz GA, et al. Risk of symptomatic gallstones in women with severe obesity. Am J Clin Nutr 1992;55:652–8.

23. Tsai CJ, Leitzmann MF, Willett WC, et al. The effect of long-term intake of cis unsaturated fats on the risk for gallstone disease in men: a prospective cohort study. Ann Intern Med 2004;141:514–22.

24. Calle EE, Rodriguez C, Walker-Thurmond K, et al. Overweight, obesity, and mortality from cancer in a prospectively studied cohort of U.S. adults. N Engl J Med 2003;348:1625–38.

25. Chen LY, Qiao QH, Zhang SC, et al. Metabolic syndrome and gallstone disease. World J Gastroenterol 2012;18:4215–20.

26. Warschkow R, Tarantino I, Ukegjini K, et al. Concomitant cholecystectomy during laparoscopic Roux-en-Y gastric bypass in obese patients is not justified: a meta-analysis. Obes Surg 2013;23:397–407.

27. Nagem RG, Lazaro-da-Silva A, de Oliveira RM, et al. Gallstone-related complications after Roux-en-Y gastric bypass: a prospective study. Hepatobiliary Pancreat Dis Int 2012;11:630–5.

28. Krishna SG, Behzadi J, Hinton A, et al. Effects of bariatric surgery on outcomes of patients with acute pancreatitis. Clin Gastroenterol Hepatol 2016;14:1001–10.e5.

29. Shiffman ML, Sugerman HJ, Kellum JM, et al. Gallstone formation after rapid weight loss: a prospective study in patients undergoing gastric bypass surgery for treatment of morbid obesity. Am J Gastroenterol 1991;86:1000–5.

30. Wudel LJ Jr, Wright JK, Debelak JP, et al. Prevention of gallstone formation in morbidly obese patients undergoing rapid weight loss: results of a randomized controlled pilot study. J Surg Res 2002;102:50–6.

31. Maclure KM, Hayes KC, Colditz GA, et al. Weight, diet, and the risk of symptomatic gallstones in middle-aged women. N Engl J Med 1989;321:563–9.

32. Freeman JB, Meyer PD, Printen KJ, et al. Analysis of gallbladder bile in morbid obesity. Am J Surg 1975;129:163–6.

33. Portincasa P, Di Ciaula A, Palmieri V, et al. Effects of cholestyramine on gallbladder and gastric emptying in obese and lean subjects. Eur J Clin Invest 1995;25:746–53.

34. Shiffman ML, Sugerman HJ, Kellum JM, et al. Changes in gallbladder bile composition following gallstone formation and weight reduction. Gastroenterology 1992;103:214–21.

35. Tsai CJ, Leitzmann MF, Willett WC, et al. Weight cycling and risk of gallstone disease in men. Arch Intern Med 2006;166:2369–74.

36. Warttig S, Ward S, Rogers G, et al. Diagnosis and management of gallstone disease: summary of NICE guidance. BMJ 2014;349:g6241.

37. Simopoulos C, Botaitis S, Karayiannakis AJ, et al. The contribution of acute chole-cystitis, obesity, and previous abdominal surgery on the outcome of laparoscopic cholecystectomy. Am Surg 2007;73:371–6.

38. Overby DW, Apelgren KN, Richardson W, et al. SAGES guidelines for the clinical application of laparoscopic biliary tract surgery. Surg Endosc 2010;24:2368–86.

39. Coupaye M, Castel B, Sami O, et al. Comparison of the incidence of cholelithiasis after sleeve gastrectomy and Roux-en-Y gastric bypass in obese patients: a pro-spective study. Surg Obes Relat Dis 2015;11:779–84.

40. Stokes CS, Gluud LL, Casper M, et al. Ursodeoxycholic acid and diets higher in fat prevent gallbladder stones during weight loss: a meta-analysis of randomized controlled trials. Clin Gastroenterol Hepatol 2014;12:1090–100.e2 [quiz: e61].

41. McNabb-Baltar J, Ravi P, Isabwe GA, et al. A population-based assessment of the burden of acute pancreatitis in the United States. Pancreas 2014;43:687–91.

42. Singla A, Simons J, Li Y, et al. Admission volume determines outcome for patients with acute pancreatitis. Gastroenterology 2009;137:1995–2001.

43. Brown A, Young B, Morton J, et al. Are health related outcomes in acute pancre-atitis improving? An analysis of national trends in the U.S. from 1997 to 2003. JOP 2008;9:408–14.

44. Banks PA, Bollen TL, Dervenis C, et al. Classification of acute pancreatitis–2012: revision of the Atlanta classification and definitions by international consensus. Gut 2013;62:102–11.

45. Yashima Y, Isayama H, Tsujino T, et al. A large volume of visceral adipose tissue leads to severe acute pancreatitis. J Gastroenterol 2011;46:1213–8.

46. Sadr-Azodi O, Orsini N, Andren-Sandberg A, et al. Abdominal and total adiposity and the risk of acute pancreatitis: a population-based prospective cohort study. Am J Gastroenterol 2013;108:133–9.

47. Martinez J, Johnson CD, Sanchez-Paya J, et al. Obesity is a definitive risk factor of severity and mortality in acute pancreatitis: an updated meta-analysis. Pan-creatology 2006;6:206–9.

48. Hong S, Qiwen B, Ying J, et al. Body mass index and the risk and prognosis of acute pancreatitis: a meta-analysis. Eur J Gastroenterol Hepatol 2011;23:1136–43.

49. Suazo-Barahona J, Carmona-Sanchez R, Robles-Diaz G, et al. Obesity: a risk factor for severe acute biliary and alcoholic pancreatitis. Am J Gastroenterol 1998;93:1324–8.

50. Porter K, Banks P. Obesity as a predictor of severity in acute pancreatitis. Int J Pancreatol 1991;10:247–52.

51. Tsai CJ. Is obesity a significant prognostic factor in acute pancreatitis? Dig Dis Sci 1998;43:2251–4.

52. De Waele B, Vanmierlo B, Van Nieuwenhove Y, et al. Impact of body overweight and class I, II and III obesity on the outcome of acute biliary pancreatitis. Pancreas 2006;32:343–5.

53. Frossard JL, Lescuyer P, Pastor CM. Experimental evidence of obesity as a risk factor for severe acute pancreatitis. World J Gastroenterol 2009;15:5260–5.

54. Wang SQ, Li SJ, Feng QX, et al. Overweight is an additional prognostic factor in acute pancreatitis: a meta-analysis. Pancreatology 2011;11:92–8.

55. Meining A, Shah RJ, Slivka A, et al. Classification of probe-based confocal laser endomicroscopy findings in pancreaticobiliary strictures. Endoscopy 2012;44:251–7.

56. Taguchi M, Kubo T, Yamamoto M, et al. Body mass index influences the outcome of acute pancreatitis: an analysis based on the Japanese administrative database. Pancreas 2014;43:863–6.

57. Saisho Y, Butler AE, Meier JJ, et al. Pancreas volumes in humans from birth to age one hundred taking into account sex, obesity, and presence of type-2 diabetes. Clin Anat 2007;20:933–42.

58. Acharya C, Cline RA, Jaligama D, et al. Fibrosis reduces severity of acute-on-chronic pancreatitis in humans. Gastroenterology 2013;145:466–75.

59. Navina S, Acharya C, DeLany JP, et al. Lipotoxicity causes multisystem organ failure and exacerbates acute pancreatitis in obesity. Sci Transl Med 2011;3:107ra110.

60. Acharya C, Navina S, Singh VP. Role of pancreatic fat in the outcomes of pancreatitis. Pancreatology 2014;14:403–8.

61. Freeman ML, Werner J, van Santvoort HC, et al. Interventions for necrotizing pancreatitis: summary of a multidisciplinary consensus conference. Pancreas 2012;41:1176–94.

62. Noel P, Patel K, Durgampudi C, et al. Peripancreatic fat necrosis worsens acute pancreatitis independent of pancreatic necrosis via unsaturated fatty acids increased in human pancreatic necrosis collections. Gut 2016;65:100–11.

63. Viana EC, Araujo-Dasilio KL, Miguel GP, et al. Gastric bypass and sleeve gastrectomy: the same impact on IL-6 and TNF-alpha. Prospective clinical trial. Obes Surg 2013;23:1252–61.

64. Rao SR. Inflammatory markers and bariatric surgery: a meta-analysis. Inflamm Res 2012;61:789–807.

65. Miller GD, Nicklas BJ, Fernandez A. Serial changes in inflammatory biomarkers after Roux-en-Y gastric bypass surgery. Surg Obes Relat Dis 2011;7:618–24.

66. Moreau JA, Zinsmeister AR, Melton LJ 3rd, et al. Gallstone pancreatitis and the effect of cholecystectomy: a population-based cohort study. Mayo Clin Proc 1988;63:466–73.

67. Kumaravel A, Zelisko A, Schauer P, et al. Acute pancreatitis in patients after bariatric surgery: incidence, outcomes, and risk factors. Obes Surg 2014;24:2025–30.

68. Rapp K, Schroeder J, Klenk J, et al. Obesity and incidence of cancer: a large cohort study of over 145,000 adults in Austria. Br J Cancer 2005;93:1062–7.

69. Li D, Morris JS, Liu J, et al. Body mass index and risk, age of onset, and survival in patients with pancreatic cancer. JAMA 2009;301:2553–62.

70. Rollins KE, Tewari N, Ackner A, et al. The impact of sarcopenia and myosteatosis on outcomes of unresectable pancreatic cancer or distal cholangiocarcinoma. Clin Nutr 2015. [Epub ahead of print].

71. Larsson SC, Permert J, Hakansson N, et al. Overall obesity, abdominal adiposity, diabetes and cigarette smoking in relation to the risk of pancreatic cancer in two Swedish population-based cohorts. Br J Cancer 2005;93:1310–5.

72. Calle EE, Kaaks R. Overweight, obesity and cancer: epidemiological evidence and proposed mechanisms. Nat Rev Cancer 2004;4:579–91.

73. Pecorelli N, Carrara G, De Cobelli F, et al. Effect of sarcopenia and visceral obesity on mortality and pancreatic fistula following pancreatic cancer surgery. Br J Surg 2016;103:434–42.

74. Tan BH, Birdsell LA, Martin L, et al. Sarcopenia in an overweight or obese patient is an adverse prognostic factor in pancreatic cancer. Clin Cancer Res 2009;15:6973–9.

75. Stolzenberg-Solomon RZ, Schairer C, Moore S, et al. Lifetime adiposity and risk of pancreatic cancer in the NIH-AARP Diet and Health Study cohort. Am J Clin Nutr 2013;98:1057–65.
76. Bethea TN, Kitahara CM, Sonderman J, et al. A pooled analysis of body mass index and pancreatic cancer mortality in african americans. Cancer Epidemiol Biomarkers Prev 2014;23:2119–25.
77. Genkinger JM, Spiegelman D, Anderson KE, et al. A pooled analysis of 14 cohort studies of anthropometric factors and pancreatic cancer risk. Int J Cancer 2011; 129:1708–17.
78. Aune D, Greenwood DC, Chan DS, et al. Body mass index, abdominal fatness and pancreatic cancer risk: a systematic review and non-linear dose-response meta-analysis of prospective studies. Ann Oncol 2012;23:843–52.
79. Genkinger JM, Kitahara CM, Bernstein L, et al. Central adiposity, obesity during early adulthood, and pancreatic cancer mortality in a pooled analysis of cohort studies. Ann Oncol 2015;26:2257–66.
80. Buchler MW, Wagner M, Schmied BM, et al. Changes in morbidity after pancreatic resection: toward the end of completion pancreatectomy. Arch Surg 2003; 138:1310–4 [discussion: 1315].
81. You L, Zhao W, Hong X, et al. The effect of body mass index on surgical outcomes in patients undergoing pancreatic resection: a systematic review and meta-analysis. Pancreas 2016;45:796–805.
82. House MG, Fong Y, Arnaoutakis DJ, et al. Preoperative predictors for complications after pancreaticoduodenectomy: impact of BMI and body fat distribution. J Gastrointest Surg 2008;12:270–8.
83. Sandini M, Bernasconi DP, Fior D, et al. A high visceral adipose tissue-to-skeletal muscle ratio as a determinant of major complications after pancreatoduodenectomy for cancer. Nutrition 2016. [Epub ahead of print].
84. Philip B, Roland CL, Daniluk J, et al. A high-fat diet activates oncogenic Kras and COX2 to induce development of pancreatic ductal adenocarcinoma in mice. Gastroenterology 2013;145:1449–58.
85. Dawson DW, Hertzer K, Moro A, et al. High-fat, high-calorie diet promotes early pancreatic neoplasia in the conditional KrasG12D mouse model. Cancer Prev Res (Phila) 2013;6:1064–73.
86. Khasawneh J, Schulz MD, Walch A, et al. Inflammation and mitochondrial fatty acid beta-oxidation link obesity to early tumor promotion. Proc Natl Acad Sci U S A 2009;106:3354–9.
87. Lashinger LM, Harrison LM, Rasmussen AJ, et al. Dietary energy balance modulation of Kras- and Ink4a/Arf+/–driven pancreatic cancer: the role of insulin-like growth factor-I. Cancer Prev Res (Phila) 2013;6:1046–55.
88. Yachida S, Jones S, Bozic I, et al. Distant metastasis occurs late during the genetic evolution of pancreatic cancer. Nature 2010;467:1114–7.

Nonalcoholic Fatty Liver Disease

Pathophysiology and Management

Rotonya M. Carr, MD*, Amanke Oranu, MD,
Vandana Khungar, MD, MSc

KEYWORDS

- Nonalcoholic fatty liver disease • NASH • Obesity • Hepatic steatosis
- NASH therapeutics • Lipid droplet • Perilipins

KEY POINTS

- Nonalcoholic fatty liver disease (NAFLD) is a systemic disease.
- NAFLD pathogenesis involves hormonal, nutritional, and genetic factors.
- NAFLD mortality is caused by cardiovascular disease, cancer, and hepatic disease.
- Patients with NAFLD should be risk stratified at diagnosis and longitudinally for the presence and degree of fibrosis, and referred if advanced disease is suspected.
- The cornerstone of NAFLD management is 7% to 9% weight loss and management of cardiovascular, oncologic, and hepatic risk factors.

INTRODUCTION

Nonalcoholic fatty liver disease (NAFLD) is a clinical diagnosis that includes the presence of 5% or more hepatic steatosis as determined by liver imaging or biopsy in the absence of secondary causes of hepatic fat accumulation (**Table 1**). NAFLD spans the spectrum of simple steatosis or nonalcoholic fatty liver (NAFL) to nonalcoholic steatohepatitis (NASH), which is defined histologically as hepatic steatosis, hepatic inflammation, and hepatocellular ballooning with or without fibrosis. NASH can progress to cirrhosis and hepatocellular carcinoma (HCC).[1]

Current estimates are that NAFLD affects 30% of the United States population; 32% of the Middle East population; 30% of the South American population; 27% of Asian

Disclosures: Research support from Intercept (R.M. Carr); NIH/NIAAA K08-AA021424, Robert Wood Johnson Foundation, Harold Amos Medical Faculty Development Award, 7158, IDOM DRC Pilot Award P30 DK019525 (R.M. Carr); and NIH/NIDDK T32 DK007066 (A. Oranu). This work was supported in part by NIH P30-DK050306, its core facilities, and its pilot grant program.
Division of Gastroenterology and Hepatology, University of Pennsylvania, Philadelphia, PA, USA
* Corresponding author. 421 Curie Boulevard, 907 Biomedical Research Building, Philadelphia, PA 19104.
E-mail address: Rotonya.Carr@uphs.upenn.edu

Table 1
Known causes of secondary hepatic steatosis

Macrovesicular Steatosis	Microvesicular Steatosis
Excessive alcohol consumption	Reye syndrome
Viral infection: hepatitis C	Viral infection delta hepatitis
Wilson disease	HELLP syndrome
Autoimmune hepatitis	Acute fatty liver of pregnancy
Parenteral nutrition	Medications (eg, valproate, tetracycline, antiretroviral)
Medications (eg, amiodarone, methotrexate, tamoxifen, corticosteroids, antiretrovirals)	Genetic anomalies and inborn errors of metabolism[a]
Starvation: Kwashiorkor	Jamaican vomiting sickness
Lipodystrophy	
Abetalipoproteinemia	

Abbreviation: HELLP, hemolysis elevated liver enzymes, low platelet count.
  [a] Lecithin–cholesterol acyltransferase deficiency, urea cycle defects, cholesterol ester storage diseases, defects of fatty acid beta oxidation, lysosomal acid lipase deficiency, and Alpers syndrome.

populations (highest in east Asians); 24% of the European population; and 13% of the African population.[2–4] In the United States, men are disproportionately affected.[5] Hispanic Americans have a higher prevalence of NAFLD compared with white people; whereas African Americans have the lowest prevalence among all racial and ethnic groups in the United States.[6] Among the Hispanic population, those of Mexican heritage have the highest prevalence, whereas Dominican Republicans have the lowest prevalence.[7,8] The cause of this racial and ethnic disparity is likely multifactorial and includes contributions from genetic, behavioral, and socioeconomic factors.[9]

NAFLD prevalence parallels that of the obesity epidemic and in the United States is expected to become the leading cause of end-stage liver disease by 2020.[10] Like patients with obesity, patients with NAFLD have a higher risk of diabetes, cardiovascular disease, and carcinoma.[11] The metabolic syndrome (defined as the presence of 3 or more of fasting glucose $\geq$100 mg/dL, blood pressure $\geq$130/85 mm Hg, triglyceride level $\geq$150 mg/dL, high-density lipoprotein cholesterol level <40 mg/dL in men or <50 mg/dL in women, waist circumference >100 cm [40 inches] in men or 88 cm [35 inches] in women[12] and if Asian American >88 cm in men or >80 cm [32 inches] in women[13]) is common in patients with NAFLD. Consequently, NAFLD is often considered its hepatic manifestation[14] (although this has recently been challenged).[15]

PATHOGENESIS

NAFLD is a metabolic disorder, and its pathogenesis involves the complex interaction among hormonal, nutritional, and genetic factors (**Fig. 1**).

Role of Hormones

Most patients with NAFLD have obesity resulting from an imbalance between high energy intake (overnutrition) and energy expenditure. Overnutrition of both high-fat foods and sugars has been linked with activating opioid and dopamine receptors in the nucleus accumbens,[16,17] an area of the brain responsible for the development of cravings. In addition, the macronutrient fructose increases cerebral blood flow to areas of the brain responsible for motivation and reward, failing to reduce satiety compared with glucose.[18] Although these pathways have not been examined specifically in NAFLD, it is conceivable that they contribute to obesity in patients with NAFLD as well. Concomitant with the activation of reward centers in response to certain

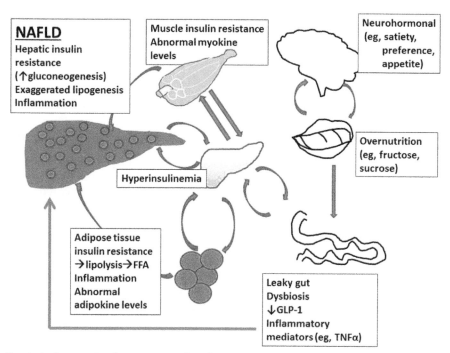

Fig. 1. Pathogenesis of NAFLD. FFA, free fatty acids; GLP-1, glucagonlike peptide 1; TNFα, tumor necrosis factor alpha.

macronutrients is the systemic reduction in levels of gut-derived hormones that promote satiety (eg, glucagonlike peptide 1 [GLP-1])[18,19] and increase in levels of gut-derived hormones that stimulate hunger (eg, ghrelin).[19] These changes are associated with an increase in circulating triglyceride levels[19] and thus are implicated in NAFLD pathogenesis.

In addition to gut-derived hormones, the adipose-derived hormones leptin and adiponectin are suspected to play a role in NAFLD pathogenesis. Leptin primarily acts centrally to reduce food intake and increase energy expenditure.[20] Adiponectin increases hepatic insulin sensitivity and reduces body fat.[21] Leptin levels are increased in patients with NAFLD, suggesting a possible contribution of leptin resistance,[22] whereas adiponectin levels are low and independently predict risk of NASH in obese patients.[23]

The systemic effects of hormones on both lipid and glucose homeostasis have inspired clinical studies investigating their efficacy in patients with NASH. For example, NASH resolved in 39% of patients who received the GLP-1 agonist liraglutide compared with 9% of patients who received placebo. Liraglutide also reduced fibrosis progression,[24] showing that hormones may be exploited to influence NAFLD risk and severity.

Role of Nutrition and Intestinal Dysbiosis

One common link among the aforementioned hormones is their regulation by nutritional status. However, because of the inherent challenges of human nutrition studies, the degree to which specific macronutrients increase NAFLD susceptibility is unknown. High-saturated-fat, low-fiber, and carbohydrate-rich diets have all been associated with NAFLD risk,[25–28] but little direct evidence exists in humans. Data from preclinical studies show that diets high in sucrose and fructose are steatogenic, perhaps through their promotion of intestinal dysbiosis or dysregulation of key lipid metabolic pathways and hormones.[29] In support of these data are studies showing that high-fructose diet[30] and high soda intake (and therefore consumption of high-fructose corn syrup)[31] increase risk of NAFLD in humans. However, such studies are based on dietary intake surveys and are unable to make direct connections between nutrient intake and NAFLD.

Microbiota are primary nutrient sensors within the gastrointestinal tract, and diet modulates gut bacterial composition in patients with NAFLD.[32] Emerging evidence shows that patients with NASH have disrupted gut epithelial tight junctions through which bacteria gain access to the systemic circulation and release inflammatory cytokines to promote hepatic steatosis and inflammation.[33,34] Investigations regarding how specific macronutrients promote these disruptions are needed to inform dietary recommendations for patients with NAFLD.

Role of Insulin Resistance, Lipotoxicity, and Hepatic Inflammation

Both hyperinsulinemia and insulin resistance are central to NAFLD pathophysiology.[35] Under normal conditions, pancreatic beta cells secrete insulin primarily in response to circulating glucose levels. Insulin acts on several metabolic tissues, including adipose tissue, to promote esterification of fatty acids and storage into lipid droplets while inhibiting the opposing process of lipolysis. In hepatocytes, insulin has 3 primary actions: to promote glycogen storage, inhibit gluconeogenesis, and activate key regulators of de novo lipogenesis. In patients with NAFLD, the development of insulin resistance results in (1) increased adipocyte lipolysis and high levels of circulating free fatty acids available for subsequent hepatic uptake, (2) reduced hepatic glycogen storage, and (3) increased gluconeogenesis. Perhaps in response to systemic insulin resistance (or preceding the development of insulin resistance[36]), hyperinsulinemia develops, which augments hepatic de novo lipogenesis pathways. The net effect is increased intrahepatic lipid accumulation (steatosis) and accentuated triglyceride secretion in the form of very-low-density lipoprotein. The increased lipid load circulates to adipose tissue, thus compounding the already reduced ability of adipocytes to store these lipids in lipid droplets.

In hepatocytes, the inability to accommodate neutral lipids within lipid droplets exposes cells to lipotoxic bioactive lipids. Lipotoxicity further impairs insulin signaling, causes oxidative damage, and promotes inflammation and fibrosis through several mechanisms.[37] These downstream effects are thought to be responsible for progression from NAFL to NASH and development of fibrosis and HCC in patients with NAFLD.

Role of Genes

Perhaps the most compelling evidence for genetic contributions to NAFLD is the observation by Makkonen and colleagues[38] that, among monozygotic Finnish twins, liver fat and serum alanine aminotransferase (ALT) levels vary independently of obesity and alcohol use. These early genetic studies have been bolstered by results from present day genome-wide association studies (GWASs) that have implicated several genetic polymorphisms associated with NAFLD risk and severity (**Table 2**). The earliest and most widely reported association is the patatin-like phospholipase domain–containing 3 (PNPLA3) gene, a protein with both triacylglycerol lipase and acylglycerol transacylase activity.[39,40] The single-nucleotide polymorphism (SNP) I148M (isoleucine to methionine at position 148) of PNPLA3 has been associated

Table 2
Genetic polymorphisms associated with NAFLD

Gene Polymorphism	Function of Gene	NAFLD Association
PNPLA3 (I148M)	Triacylglycerol lipase, acylglycerol transacylase	Increases NAFLD risk and severity; highest prevalence in Hispanic Americans (highest in Mexican Americans)[42,45,49,50]
PNPLA3 (S453I)	Triacylglycerol lipase, acylglycerol transacylase	Reduces NAFLD risk and severity; highest prevalence in African Americans[42]
NCAN	Cell adhesion molecule	Hepatic steatosis, liver inflammation, and fibrosis[45,49,84]
GCKR	Glucokinase inhibitor	Hepatic steatosis, increased ALT level[45,49]
TM6SF2 (E167K)	Unknown	Increased ALT, AST, and hepatic fat levels, small effect size[85]
PPP1R3B	Hepatic glycogen synthesis	Hepatic steatosis[45,49,50]

Abbreviations: GCKR, glucokinase regulatory protein; NCAN, neurocan; PNPLA3, patatin-like phospholipase domain-containing 3; PPP1R3B, protein phosphatase 1 regulatory subunit 3B; TM6SF2; transmembrane 6-superfamily member 2.

with both NAFLD risk and severity in adults[41–43] and children.[44] This so-called G allele is found most commonly among Hispanic people and least frequently among African Americans,[42] the demographic groups with the highest and lowest risk of NAFLD in the US population, respectively. Among Hispanic people, Mexican Americans have the highest prevalence of the G allele.[45] In contrast, a serine to isoleucine change in codon 453 seems to be protective of hepatic steatosis and is most commonly seen in African Americans.[42] Whether PNPLA3 per se is involved pathogenically in NAFLD is still unclear owing partially to inconsistencies in cell culture and in vivo genetic models.[46–48]

GWASs have identified several additional loci associated with NAFLD, namely neurocan (NCAN), glucokinase regulator (GCKR), lysophospholipaselike 1 (LYPLAL1), transmembrane 6-superfamily member 2 (TM6SF2), and protein phosphatase 1 regulatory subunit 3B (PPP1R3B).[45,49] Like PNPLA3 polymorphisms, these genes have differential associations with ethnic groups[50] and together are estimated to account for as much as 28% of the variation in hepatic steatosis as measured by computed tomography (CT) scan.[49] A summary of these genes is included in **Table 2**. The functional significance of all of these genes has not been fully determined in patients with NAFLD, thus highlighting some of the challenges inherent in extrapolating GWAS data to clinical care and showing the limitations of using these tools in whole-population screens.

DIAGNOSIS AND STAGING
Noninvasive Tests

Diagnosis of NAFLD is based on a combination of clinical factors and liver imaging. Clinical assessment involves a detailed alcohol consumption history, examination of personal and family metabolic risk factors, medication history (including supplements), and serologic testing. A summary of our approach to initial evaluation is outlined in **Table 3**.

Liver enzymes are not a component of NAFLD diagnostic criteria, as up to 60% of patients with NAFLD with normal ALT can have NASH or advanced fibrosis, and 53% of patients with NAFLD with increased ALT do not have NASH or advanced fibrosis.[51,52]

Table 3
Initial evaluation of a patient with suspected NAFLD

History	Physical Examination	Serology
Patterns of weight loss and weight gain; antiobesity interventions	Blood pressure, weight, height (calculate BMI)	Hepatic and basic metabolic panel (for creatinine)
Dietary and exercise patterns	Distribution of obesity	CBC
Alcohol intake	Stigmata of insulin resistance (eg, acanthosis nigricans)	INR
Use of parenteral nutrition	Stigmata of hypertriglyceridemia (eg, xanthomas)	Fasting lipids
Fertility history, menstrual history		Fasting glucose, insulin (calculate HOMA-IR), HbA1C
Risk factors for viral hepatitis	Stigmata of chronic liver disease (eg, icterus, jaundice, ascites, spider angiomata, palmar erythema)	Hepatitis C virus antibody
History of autoimmune diseases or suggestive symptoms		ANA and iron panel Other[a] (eg, additional autoantibody titers, ceruloplasmin, alpha 1 antitrypsin, lysosomal acid lipase activity)
Review of steatogenic medications	Stigmata of primary endocrine disorder	
Family history of liver disease, obesity, diabetes, hyperlipidemia, cardiovascular disease, cancer	Stigmata of autoimmune disease (eg, skin rashes, joint findings)	

Abbreviations: ANA, anti-nuclear antibody; BMI, body mass index; CBC, complete blood count; HbA1C, hemoglobin A1C; HOMA-IR, homeostatic model assessment-insulin resistance; INR, International Normalized Ratio.
  [a] These tests can be individualized based on patient risk factors.

Despite using the standard assessments, diagnosis of NAFLD remains challenging in some patients because high serum autoantibody, high ferritin, and low ceruloplasmin levels can be seen in the absence of concomitant chronic liver disease. As many as 20% of patients with NAFLD may have abnormal autoantibody titers.[53–55] Abnormal results of serologic tests in the context of additional clinical features that support alternative diagnoses should be evaluated further and may require liver biopsy.

Clinical history and serologic testing are combined with radiologic findings (ultrasonography, CT, or MRI) to make the diagnosis of NAFLD in most patients. Notably, most patients diagnosed with NAFLD are initially suspected because of an incidental radiologic finding of hepatic steatosis. The presence of at least 30% hepatic steatosis is optimal to visualize hepatic steatosis by these common radiology tools,[56] although there is wide interobserver and intraobserver variability.[57] None of the standard radiologic modalities can detect the presence of steatohepatitis or early fibrosis.[57]

The inability of standard radiology protocols to detect advanced stages of NAFLD has spurred research in other noninvasive strategies to stage NAFLD severity. Serologic tests and biomarker panels, ultrasound transient elastography (TE), and MRI elastography (MRE) can be used to stage NAFLD. Cytokeratin-18 (CK-18) is a hepatocyte intermediate filament that is cleaved by caspases during apoptosis and whose serum levels are increased in patients with NASH.[58] Although this test discriminates NAFL from NASH, CK-18 is not commercially available in the United States, thus limiting its practical use. Unlike discrimination of NASH, several modalities are available for the noninvasive assessment of fibrosis in patients with NAFLD. The most validated biomarker panel is the NAFLD Fibrosis Score (NFS),[1] which calculates the probability of advanced fibrosis based on readily available clinical data: age, body mass index, aspartate transaminase (AST), ALT, platelets, albumin, and presence or absence of impaired fasting glucose. A low cutoff score (−1.455) excludes advanced fibrosis (negative predictive value of 93%), whereas a high cutoff score (0.676) suggests advanced fibrosis (positive predictive value 90%).[59]

Both TE and MRE measure liver stiffness. TE performs less well in obese patients, with a failure rate of up to 16%,[60] and overestimates fibrosis in patients with significant steatosis or inflammation.[61] An extralarge (XL) probe for TE was designed for use in overweight and obese patients; however, median liver stiffness measurements were lower with the XL probe compared with the standard medium (M) probe.[62] To date, these differences have not resulted in a new scoring system with use of this probe limiting interpretation of XL probe–derived results. MRE performs better than TE for fibrosis assessment[63] but the expense of this technology limits widespread adoption.

Liver Biopsy

Because of the limitations of noninvasive testing in patients with NAFLD, liver biopsy remains the gold standard for NAFLD staging. Nevertheless, the prevalence of NAFLD, low likelihood of progressive disease in most patients, dearth of treatment options, risk of biopsy, and the uncertain cost-effectiveness of invasive testing preclude liver biopsy from being recommended in all patients. Current guidelines limit liver biopsy to those patients who have an uncertain diagnosis or who are likely to have advanced disease based on the noninvasive assessment modalities described earlier.[1] Consensus guidelines recommend the use of a transjugular approach for patients who are morbidly obese with an obscured flank site. To reduce risk of bleeding, guidelines recommend the following[64]:

- Hold antiplatelets from several days to 10 days prior
- Hold warfarin at least 5 days prior
- Hold heparin products 12 to 24 hours prior
- Weigh the above against risk of thrombotic event

Although there is no formal recommendation regarding the use of vitamin E before liver biopsy, vitamin E in high doses has anticoagulant properties[65] and consideration may be made to hold this before liver biopsy.

The range of NAFLD histology includes simple steatosis, steatohepatitis, fibrosis, and cirrhosis. Of these, fibrosis is the histologic feature that best predicts NAFLD mortality.[66] Steatosis results from hepatocellular accumulation of cytoplasmic macrovesicular lipid droplets that displace the nucleus. Lipid droplets are cores of primarily neutral lipids (triglycerides) surrounded by a single phospholipid membrane. The membrane is composed of lipid droplet proteins and metabolically active enzymes. The predominant hepatocellular lipid droplet proteins are members of the perilipin family of proteins. Perilipin 2 and perilipin 3 are expressed in NAFL whereas perilipin 1 is de novo expressed in steatohepatitis.[67–70]

The recent NASH Clinical Research Network pathologic scoring system is based on the original Brunt histologic criteria but expands the fibrosis stages to delineate pattern of fibrosis.[71] Even with expert pathology examination, challenges remain with staging patients with NAFLD. Because a standard needle biopsy sample approximates only 0.00002 of the mass of the liver,[64] liver biopsy specimens are highly variable,[72] which underscores the need for providers to be judicious in recommending liver biopsy for the management of patients with NAFLD.

MANAGEMENT

Mortality from NAFLD is caused by cardiometabolic disease (12.7%), non-HCC malignancy (8.1%), and liver disease (including HCC) (6.9%).[11] Eighteen-year liver-related mortality is greater in NASH compared with patients without NASH (17.5% vs 2.7%, respectively).[11] The risk of mortality from cardiometabolic and oncologic disease in patients with NAFLD requires that special attention be paid to both metabolic and cancer risk factors; namely assessment and management of obesity, hyperlipidemia (notwithstanding institution of statins, which improve mortality in cirrhotic patients with NASH[66]), insulin resistance, and diabetes is recommended for all patients. In addition, patients are advised to undergo standard cancer screening examinations according to their age, gender, and family history. In our practice, we additionally comanage patients with primary care, cardiology, endocrinology, and nutrition (**Table 4**).

In addition to surveillance of risk factors for mortality, all patients should be placed on an appropriate dietary and exercise regimen to promote weight loss of at least 5% for those with NAFL or 7% to 9% for those with NASH. Such lifestyle modification improves transaminase levels and liver histology[73] and also reverses fibrosis[74]; 90% of patients who achieve greater than or equal to 10% weight loss have complete NASH resolution.[74]

The finding of advanced fibrosis or cirrhosis on liver biopsy in a patient with NAFLD necessitates screening for complications of cirrhosis and referral to hepatology if a referral has not already been made. In addition to standard dietary recommendations, the authors recommend complete alcohol abstinence for patients with advanced NAFLD. All patients with advanced fibrosis and cirrhosis require both endoscopic variceal screening and radiologic surveillance for HCC every 6 months. There may be an increased risk of HCC even in the absence of cirrhosis in NAFLD. Among patients with metabolic syndrome and no other cause of chronic liver disease, 65.5% of patients with HCC had no or mild fibrosis, and patients diagnosed with cryptogenic cirrhosis without apparent metabolic syndrome developed HCC in nonfibrotic livers more commonly than in fibrotic livers (75% vs 25%).[75] Further studies are warranted to determine the feasibility and utility of earlier HCC screening in patients with NAFLD.

Approved Pharmacologic Therapy and Investigational Agents

Only 2 therapies are currently recommended for use in patients with NASH: pioglitazone and vitamin E. In both diabetic[76] and nondiabetic patients,[77] treatment with pioglitazone (30–45 mg daily) improves NASH compared with placebo.[77] However, treatment is associated with significant weight gain. Vitamin E was investigated in the PIVENS (pioglitazone or vitamin E vs placebo in nondiabetic patients with NASH) trial. Patients treated with 800 IU of vitamin E daily for 96 weeks showed reduced steatosis and inflammation.[77] The use of vitamin E is reserved for biopsy-proven NASH in nondiabetic patients.

Table 4
Strategies to reduce cardiovascular (CV), oncologic, and hepatic mortality in patients with NAFLD

CV	Oncologic	Hepatic
• Glycemic control	• Glycemic control	• Glycemic control
• Weight loss	• Weight loss	• Weight loss
• Lipid level lowering	• Assess cancer risk	• Minimize/avoid alcohol
• Collaborate with cardiology, endocrinology	• Offer routine screening	• ±Rx
		• Variceal and HCC screening (if advanced disease)

Abbreviation: Rx, pharmacologic.

Investigational Therapies

Over the past several years, there has been a surge in NAFLD therapeutic trials. Among the investigational agents is a new class of farnesoid X receptor (FXR) agonists. FXR agonists regulate both glucose and lipid homeostasis. Obeticholic acid is the first drug in this class under investigation for NASH.[78] A recent randomized, double-blinded, placebo-controlled trial of nondiabetic patients with NASH showed improvement in histologic NASH in 45% of patients who received obeticholic acid versus 21% of patients who received placebo. In addition, patients who received obeticholic acid had improvement of fibrosis compared with placebo.[79] There was a lack of improvement in insulin sensitivity and dyslipidemia that developed in patients who took obeticholic acid, and a phase III trial is currently underway.[80]

The peroxisome proliferator-activated receptors (PPAR)α/δ agent elafibranor has also recently been studied in NASH. Compared with placebo, elafibranor improved liver enzyme and serum lipid levels. In an intention-to-treat analysis of the primary end point, elafibranor failed to resolve NASH; however, using a modified end point, elafibranor resolved NASH without fibrosis worsening (20% vs 11%). This medication caused a reversible increase in serum creatinine level and, as a result, requires further investigation.[81]

Besides pharmacotherapy, several studies have shown the effectiveness of obesity surgery for NASH, showing up to 85% NASH resolution 1 year after surgery.[82] Although there are now several antiobesity endoscopic procedures under investigation,[83] none have been evaluated for the primary indication of NASH. However, it is conceivable that there would be improvements in NASH histology if similar weight loss is achieved with these procedures.

Regardless of the modality, the management of patients with NAFLD requires interventions that work systemically to integrate hepatic and extrahepatic signals. Such therapies must incorporate lifestyle changes to affect cardiovascular end points and accomplish weight reduction because weight loss of 7% to 10% is currently the only therapy that achieves NASH resolution in most patients.

SUMMARY

NAFLD is an important cause of morbidity and mortality worldwide because of both cardiovascular and oncologic sequelae as well as because it is rapidly becoming the leading cause of end-stage liver disease and liver transplant. With a prevalence of 30% in the United States it has reached epidemic proportions. Although the metabolic syndrome is a common risk factor, there are differences among racial and ethnic groups, suggesting the complex interaction between hormonal, nutritional, and genetic factors at play in disease pathogenesis. Furthermore, these biological factors likely intersect with socioeconomic forces that ultimately influence people's susceptibility to NAFLD and likelihood of progression to advanced stages.

The complexity of NAFLD pathogenesis mirrors that of its management in that successful care of patients with NAFLD requires a multisystem, integrated approach. Close attention must be paid to overall metabolic health in addition to hepatic health. Providers should assess and manage risk factors aggressively and estimate risk of fibrosis at presentation and longitudinally. Hepatology referral can be made at any stage but especially at the stage at which fibrosis is suspected. The arena of treatment options is an area ripe for innovation because few currently approved treatments exist. Regression of NASH and fibrosis is possible with weight loss; however, the authors anticipate that adjunctive pharmacologic and nonpharmacologic therapies may be available for the care of patients with NAFLD in the future.

REFERENCES

1. Chalasani N, Younossi Z, Lavine JE, et al. The diagnosis and management of non-alcoholic fatty liver disease: practice guideline by the American Association for the Study of Liver Diseases, American College of Gastroenterology, and the American Gastroenterological Association. Hepatology 2012;55:2005–23.
2. Younossi ZM, Koenig AB, Abdelatif D, et al. Global epidemiology of nonalcoholic fatty liver disease–Meta-analytic assessment of prevalence, incidence and outcomes. Hepatology 2015;64:73–84.
3. Vernon G, Baranova A, Younossi ZM. Systematic review: the epidemiology and natural history of non-alcoholic fatty liver disease and non-alcoholic steatohepatitis in adults. Aliment Pharmacol Ther 2011;34:274–85.
4. Petersen KF, Dufour S, Feng J, et al. Increased prevalence of insulin resistance and nonalcoholic fatty liver disease in Asian-Indian men. Proc Natl Acad Sci U S A 2006;103:18273–7.
5. Pan JJ, Fallon MB. Gender and racial differences in nonalcoholic fatty liver disease. World J Hepatol 2014;6:274–83.
6. Browning JD, Szczepaniak LS, Dobbins R, et al. Prevalence of hepatic steatosis in an urban population in the United States: impact of ethnicity. Hepatology 2004;40:1387–95.
7. Fleischman MW, Budoff M, Zeb I, et al. NAFLD prevalence differs among Hispanic subgroups: the multi-ethnic study of atherosclerosis. World J Gastroenterol 2014;20:4987–93.
8. Kallwitz ER, Daviglus ML, Allison MA, et al. Prevalence of suspected nonalcoholic fatty liver disease in Hispanic/Latino individuals differs by heritage. Clin Gastroenterol Hepatol 2015;13:569–76.
9. Saab S, Manne V, Nieto J, et al. Nonalcoholic fatty liver disease in Latinos. Clin Gastroenterol Hepatol 2016;14:5–12 [quiz: e9–10].
10. Charlton MR, Burns JM, Pedersen RA, et al. Frequency and outcomes of liver transplantation for nonalcoholic steatohepatitis in the united states. Gastroenterology 2011;141:1249–53.
11. Rafiq N, Bai C, Fang Y, et al. Long-term follow-up of patients with nonalcoholic fatty liver. Clin Gastroenterol Hepatol 2009;7:234–8.
12. Grundy SM, Cleeman JI, Daniels SR, et al. Diagnosis and management of the metabolic syndrome: an American Heart Association/National Heart, Lung, and Blood Institute scientific statement. Circulation 2005;112:2735–52.
13. Liu J, Grundy SM, Wang W, et al. Ethnic-specific criteria for the metabolic syndrome: evidence from china. Diabetes Care 2006;29:1414–6.
14. Marchesini G, Bugianesi E, Forlani G, et al. Nonalcoholic fatty liver, steatohepatitis, and the metabolic syndrome. Hepatology 2003;37:917–23.
15. Lonardo A, Ballestri S, Marchesini G, et al. Nonalcoholic fatty liver disease: a precursor of the metabolic syndrome. Dig Liver Dis 2015;47:181–90.
16. Pelchat ML, Johnson A, Chan R, et al. Images of desire: food-craving activation during fMRI. Neuroimage 2004;23:1486–93.
17. Kelley AE, Bakshi VP, Haber SN, et al. Opioid modulation of taste hedonics within the ventral striatum. Physiol Behav 2002;76:365–77.

18. Page KA, Chan O, Arora J, et al. Effects of fructose vs glucose on regional cerebral blood flow in brain regions involved with appetite and reward pathways. JAMA 2013;309:63–70.

19. Teff KL, Elliott SS, Tschop M, et al. Dietary fructose reduces circulating insulin and leptin, attenuates postprandial suppression of ghrelin, and increases triglycerides in women. J Clin Endocrinol Metab 2004;89:2963–72.

20. Ahima RS, Flier JS. Leptin. Annu Rev Physiol 2000;62:413–37.

21. Buechler C, Wanninger J, Neumeier M. Adiponectin, a key adipokine in obesity related liver diseases. World J Gastroenterol 2011;17:2801–11.

22. Chitturi S, Farrell G, Frost L, et al. Serum leptin in NASH correlates with hepatic steatosis but not fibrosis: a manifestation of lipotoxicity? Hepatology 2002;36: 403–9.

23. Targher G, Bertolini L, Rodella S, et al. Associations between plasma adiponectin concentrations and liver histology in patients with nonalcoholic fatty liver disease. Clin Endocrinol (Oxf) 2006;64:679–83.

24. Armstrong MJ, Gaunt P, Aithal GP, et al. Liraglutide safety and efficacy in patients with non-alcoholic steatohepatitis (LEAN): a multicentre, double-blind, randomised, placebo-controlled phase 2 study. Lancet 2016;387:679–90.

25. Kang H, Greenson JK, Omo JT, et al. Metabolic syndrome is associated with greater histologic severity, higher carbohydrate, and lower fat diet in patients with NAFLD. Am J Gastroenterol 2006;101:2247–53.

26. Musso G, Gambino R, De Michieli F, et al. Dietary habits and their relations to insulin resistance and postprandial lipemia in nonalcoholic steatohepatitis. Hepatology 2003;37:909–16.

27. Lai HS, Lin WH, Chen PR, et al. Effects of a high-fiber diet on hepatocyte apoptosis and liver regeneration after partial hepatectomy in rats with fatty liver. JPEN J Parenter Enteral Nutr 2005;29:401–7.

28. Sullivan S. Implications of diet on nonalcoholic fatty liver disease. Curr Opin Gastroenterol 2010;26:160–4.

29. Festi D, Schiumerini R, Eusebi LH, et al. Gut microbiota and metabolic syndrome. World J Gastroenterol 2014;20:16079–94.

30. Ouyang X, Cirillo P, Sautin Y, et al. Fructose consumption as a risk factor for nonalcoholic fatty liver disease. J Hepatol 2008;48:993–9.

31. Abid A, Taha O, Nseir W, et al. Soft drink consumption is associated with fatty liver disease independent of metabolic syndrome. J Hepatol 2009;51:918–24.

32. Mouzaki M, Comelli EM, Arendt BM, et al. Intestinal microbiota in patients with nonalcoholic fatty liver disease. Hepatology 2013;58:120–7.

33. Miele L, Valenza V, La Torre G, et al. Increased intestinal permeability and tight junction alterations in nonalcoholic fatty liver disease. Hepatology 2009;49: 1877–87.

34. Giorgio V, Miele L, Principessa L, et al. Intestinal permeability is increased in children with non-alcoholic fatty liver disease, and correlates with liver disease severity. Dig Liver Dis 2014;46:556–60.

35. Fu Z, Gilbert ER, Liu D. Regulation of insulin synthesis and secretion and pancreatic beta-cell dysfunction in diabetes. Curr Diabetes Rev 2013;9:25–53.

36. McGarry JD. What if Minkowski had been ageusic? An alternative angle on diabetes. Science 1992;258:766–70.

37. Gao B, Tsukamoto H. Inflammation in alcoholic and nonalcoholic fatty liver disease: friend or foe? Gastroenterology 2016;150:1704–9.

38. Makkonen J, Pietilainen KH, Rissanen A, et al. Genetic factors contribute to variation in serum alanine aminotransferase activity independent of obesity and alcohol: a study in monozygotic and dizygotic twins. J Hepatol 2009;50:1035–42.

39. Jenkins CM, Mancuso DJ, Yan W, et al. Identification, cloning, expression, and purification of three novel human calcium-independent phospholipase a2 family members possessing triacylglycerol lipase and acylglycerol transacylase activities. J Biol Chem 2004;279:48968–75.

40. He S, McPhaul C, Li JZ, et al. A sequence variation (I148M) in PNPLA3 associated with nonalcoholic fatty liver disease disrupts triglyceride hydrolysis. J Biol Chem 2010;285:6706–15.

41. Speliotes EK, Butler JL, Palmer CD, et al. PNPLA3 variants specifically confer increased risk for histologic nonalcoholic fatty liver disease but not metabolic disease. Hepatology 2010;52:904–12.

42. Romeo S, Kozlitina J, Xing C, et al. Genetic variation in PNPLA3 confers susceptibility to nonalcoholic fatty liver disease. Nat Genet 2008;40:1461–5.

43. Sookoian S, Pirola CJ. Meta-analysis of the influence of I148M variant of patatin-like phospholipase domain containing 3 gene (PNPLA3) on the susceptibility and histological severity of nonalcoholic fatty liver disease. Hepatology 2011;53:1883–94.

44. Santoro N, Kursawe R, D'Adamo E, et al. A common variant in the patatin-like phospholipase 3 gene (PNPLA3) is associated with fatty liver disease in obese children and adolescents. Hepatology 2010;52:1281–90.

45. Hernaez R, McLean J, Lazo M, et al. Association between variants in or near PNPLA3, GCKR, and PPP1R3B with ultrasound-defined steatosis based on data from the third National Health and Nutrition Examination Survey. Clin Gastroenterol Hepatol 2013;11:1183–90.e2.

46. Basantani MK, Sitnick MT, Cai L, et al. PNPLA3/adiponutrin deficiency in mice does not contribute to fatty liver disease or metabolic syndrome. J Lipid Res 2011;52:318–29.

47. Li JZ, Huang Y, Karaman R, et al. Chronic overexpression of PNPLA3[I148M] in mouse liver causes hepatic steatosis. J Clin Invest 2012;122:4130–44.

48. Smagris E, BasuRay S, Li J, et al. *PNPLA3I148M* knockin mice accumulate PNPLA3 on lipid droplets and develop hepatic steatosis. Hepatology 2015;61:108–18.

49. Speliotes EK, Yerges-Armstrong LM, Wu J, et al. Genome-wide association analysis identifies variants associated with nonalcoholic fatty liver disease that have distinct effects on metabolic traits. PLoS Genet 2011;7:e1001324.

50. Palmer ND, Musani SK, Yerges-Armstrong LM, et al. Characterization of European ancestry nonalcoholic fatty liver disease-associated variants in individuals of African and Hispanic descent. Hepatology 2013;58:966–75.

51. Fracanzani AL, Valenti L, Bugianesi E, et al. Risk of severe liver disease in nonalcoholic fatty liver disease with normal aminotransferase levels: a role for insulin resistance and diabetes. Hepatology 2008;48:792–8.

52. Verma S, Jensen D, Hart J, et al. Predictive value of ALT levels for non-alcoholic steatohepatitis (NASH) and advanced fibrosis in non-alcoholic fatty liver disease (NAFLD). Liver Int 2013;33:1398–405.

53. Adams LA, Lindor KD, Angulo P. The prevalence of autoantibodies and autoimmune hepatitis in patients with nonalcoholic fatty liver disease. Am J Gastroenterol 2004;99:1316–20.

54. Cotler SJ, Kanji K, Keshavarzian A, et al. Prevalence and significance of autoantibodies in patients with non-alcoholic steatohepatitis. J Clin Gastroenterol 2004; 38:801–4.
55. Loria P, Lonardo A, Leonardi F, et al. Non-organ-specific autoantibodies in nonalcoholic fatty liver disease: prevalence and correlates. Dig Dis Sci 2003;48: 2173–81.
56. Lee SS, Park SH, Kim HJ, et al. Non-invasive assessment of hepatic steatosis: prospective comparison of the accuracy of imaging examinations. J Hepatol 2010;52:579–85.
57. Saadeh S, Younossi ZM, Remer EM, et al. The utility of radiological imaging in nonalcoholic fatty liver disease. Gastroenterology 2002;123:745–50.
58. Feldstein AE, Wieckowska A, Lopez AR, et al. Cytokeratin-18 fragment levels as noninvasive biomarkers for nonalcoholic steatohepatitis: a multicenter validation study. Hepatology 2009;50:1072–8.
59. Angulo P, Hui JM, Marchesini G, et al. The NAFLD fibrosis score: a noninvasive system that identifies liver fibrosis in patients with NAFLD. Hepatology 2007;45: 846–54.
60. Castera L, Foucher J, Bernard PH, et al. Pitfalls of liver stiffness measurement: a 5-year prospective study of 13,369 examinations. Hepatology 2010;51:828–35.
61. Rinaldi L, Restivo L, Guerrera B, et al. Hepatic steatosis and necro-inflammatory activity overestimate liver stiffness by transient elastography in staging liver fibrosis in chronic hepatitis c. J Hepat Res 2014;1:1012.
62. Myers RP, Pomier-Layrargues G, Kirsch R, et al. Feasibility and diagnostic performance of the FibroScan XL probe for liver stiffness measurement in overweight and obese patients. Hepatology 2012;55:199–208.
63. Imajo K, Kessoku T, Honda Y, et al. Magnetic resonance imaging more accurately classifies steatosis and fibrosis in patients with nonalcoholic fatty liver disease than transient elastography. Gastroenterology 2016;150:626–37.e7.
64. Rockey DC, Caldwell SH, Goodman ZD, et al. Liver biopsy. Hepatology 2009;49: 1017–44.
65. Booth SL, Golly I, Sacheck JM, et al. Effect of vitamin E supplementation on vitamin K status in adults with normal coagulation status. Am J Clin Nutr 2004; 80:143–8.
66. Angulo P, Kleiner DE, Dam-Larsen S, et al. Liver fibrosis, but no other histologic features, is associated with long-term outcomes of patients with nonalcoholic fatty liver disease. Gastroenterology 2015;149:389–97.e10.
67. Carr RM, Ahima RS. Pathophysiology of lipid droplet proteins in liver diseases. Exp Cell Res 2016;340:187–92.
68. Straub BK, Gyoengyoesi B, Koenig M, et al. Adipophilin/perilipin-2 as a lipid droplet-specific marker for metabolically active cells and diseases associated with metabolic dysregulation. Histopathology 2013;62:617–31.
69. Straub BK, Stoeffel P, Heid H, et al. Differential pattern of lipid droplet-associated proteins and de novo perilipin expression in hepatocyte steatogenesis. Hepatology 2008;47:1936–46.
70. Carr RM, Patel RT, Rao V, et al. Reduction of TIP47 improves hepatic steatosis and glucose homeostasis in mice. Am J Physiol Regul Integr Comp Physiol 2012;302:R996–1003.
71. Kleiner DE, Brunt EM, Van Natta M, et al. Design and validation of a histological scoring system for nonalcoholic fatty liver disease. Hepatology 2005;41:1313–21.
72. Ratziu V, Charlotte F, Heurtier A, et al. Sampling variability of liver biopsy in nonalcoholic fatty liver disease. Gastroenterology 2005;128:1898–906.

73. Promrat K, Kleiner DE, Niemeier HM, et al. Randomized controlled trial testing the effects of weight loss on nonalcoholic steatohepatitis. Hepatology 2010;51: 121–9.

74. Vilar-Gomez E, Martinez-Perez Y, Calzadilla-Bertot L, et al. Weight loss through lifestyle modification significantly reduces features of nonalcoholic steatohepatitis. Gastroenterology 2015;149:367–78.e5 [quiz: e314–65].

75. Paradis V, Zalinski S, Chelbi E, et al. Hepatocellular carcinomas in patients with metabolic syndrome often develop without significant liver fibrosis: a pathological analysis. Hepatology 2009;49:851–9.

76. Belfort R, Harrison SA, Brown K, et al. A placebo-controlled trial of pioglitazone in subjects with nonalcoholic steatohepatitis. N Engl J Med 2006;355:2297–307.

77. Chalasani NP, Sanyal AJ, Kowdley KV, et al. Pioglitazone versus vitamin E versus placebo for the treatment of non-diabetic patients with non-alcoholic steatohepatitis: PIVENS trial design. Contemp Clin Trials 2009;30:88–96.

78. Carr RM, Reid AE. FXR agonists as therapeutic agents for non-alcoholic fatty liver disease. Curr Atheroscler Rep 2015;17:500.

79. Neuschwander-Tetri BA, Loomba R, Sanyal AJ, et al. Farnesoid X nuclear receptor ligand obeticholic acid for non-cirrhotic, non-alcoholic steatohepatitis (FLINT): a multicentre, randomised, placebo-controlled trial. Lancet 2015;385:956–65.

80. Clinical trials.Gov. 2016. Available at: https://clinicaltrials.gov/ct2/show/NCT02548351.

81. Ratziu V, Harrison SA, Francque S, et al. Elafibranor, an agonist of the peroxisome proliferator-activated receptor-alpha and -delta, induces resolution of nonalcoholic steatohepatitis without fibrosis worsening. Gastroenterology 2016;150: 1147–59.e5.

82. Lassailly G, Caiazzo R, Buob D, et al. Bariatric surgery reduces features of nonalcoholic steatohepatitis in morbidly obese patients. Gastroenterology 2015;149: 379–88 [quiz: e315–376].

83. Abu Dayyeh BK, Edmundowicz SA, Jonnalagadda S, et al. Endoscopic bariatric therapies. Gastrointest Endosc 2015;81:1073–86.

84. Gorden A, Yang R, Yerges-Armstrong LM, et al. Genetic variation at NCAN locus is associated with inflammation and fibrosis in non-alcoholic fatty liver disease in morbid obesity. Hum Hered 2013;75:34–43.

85. Sookoian S, Pirola CJ. Meta-analysis of the influence of TM6SF2 E167K variant on plasma concentration of aminotransferases across different populations and diverse liver phenotypes. Sci Rep 2016;6:27718.

Dietary and Behavioral Approaches in the Management of Obesity

Kimberly Gudzune, MD, MPH

KEYWORDS

- Obesity • Weight loss • Diet • Reducing • Weight reduction programs
- Body weight maintenance

KEY POINTS

- Clinicians should use an evidenced-based strategy like the 5As—assess, advise, agree, assist, arrange—to facilitate weight management counseling with their patients.
- Initial weight loss goal should be a 3% to 5% loss over a 3- to 6-month period through engaging in a high-intensity, comprehensive lifestyle change program that includes a moderately reduced calorie diet, increased physical activity, and behavioral strategies.
- Referral to locally available evidence-based weight loss programs should be considered, including the National Diabetes Prevention Program or commercial weight-loss programs like Weight Watchers or Jenny Craig.
- Continued follow-up and surveillance after weight loss are critical for weight loss maintenance.

INTRODUCTION

Approximately two-thirds of US adults are overweight or obese.[1] Elevated body weight has been associated with increased risk of cardiovascular disease, type 2 diabetes mellitus, kidney disease, and certain cancers[2]; however, losing weight can prevent or improve control of some obesity-related chronic conditions.[3–5] The US Preventive Services Task Force recommends high-intensity counseling interventions for individuals with obesity that include nutrition, physical activity, self-monitoring, goal setting, and group or individuals sessions.[6] In 2013, the American Heart Association, American College of Cardiology and The Obesity Society (AHA/ACC/TOS) released evidenced-based guidelines for the management of obesity among adults.[7] In this article, the clinicians' roles in weight management are discussed, particularly how to implement these guidelines and other recent advancements in dietary and behavioral approaches into clinical practice.

Conflicts of Interest: The author has none to disclose.

Department of Medicine, Johns Hopkins University School of Medicine, 2024 East Monument Street, Room 2-621, Baltimore, MD 21287, USA

E-mail address: gudzune@jhu.edu

Gastroenterol Clin N Am 45 (2016) 653–661
http://dx.doi.org/10.1016/j.gtc.2016.07.004

gastro.theclinics.com

THE CLINICIAN'S ROLE IN WEIGHT MANAGEMENT

Clinicians may assume a variety of roles in the management of obesity, varying based on their interest, education/training, and time. Prior studies of physicians have often cited a lack of training or experience regarding weight management as a major barrier to counseling their patients.[8,9] Clinicians who did not receive adequate training on obesity might consider continuing medical education in this area if they plan to take a leading role in weight management. For physicians who plan to dedicate significant clinical effort in this area, certification through the American Board of Obesity Medicine (http://www.abom.org/) or other entity might be considered. Lack of time is another common barrier to weight management.[8] Clinicians should also be aware that the recommended intensity of follow-up may require at least monthly visits with patients,[7] if not more frequently. If adequate follow-up for patients cannot be accommodated, then referral to such programs that meet this requirement should be considered. Although some physicians have reported avoiding weight loss discussions for fear of offending their patients,[10] evidence supports the clinician's role in referring patients into programs, providing accountability for patients, acting to cheerlead for patients during follow-up visits, and maintaining the long-term trusting relationship through the ups and downs of weight loss.[11]

Three key aspects—interest, training, and time—may influence the decision of whether a clinician might take a leading role in weight management or prefer the job of identifying and referring patients to appropriate weight management programs (**Box 1**). Regardless of whether the clinician decides to take an active or passive role, prior studies have documented the benefits of health care provider engagement in weight management. In a randomized controlled trial of a weight loss intervention in which clinicians referred their patients to the program, patients who rated their physicians as more helpful lost significantly more weight than those who did not rate their physicians highly.[12] When clinicians discuss weight loss without communicating judgment, patients are more likely to achieve a clinically significant weight loss.[13]

WEIGHT MANAGEMENT IN CLINICAL PRACTICE

Clinicians' key duties involve identifying appropriate patients for referral, determining the weight management strategy, and following up on patients' progress. Regardless of whether the clinician takes an active or passive role, using an evidence-based behavior change strategy, such as the 5As, assess, advise, agree, assist, arrange (**Box 2**),[14,15] can help guide assessment and counseling. Conversations that use the 5As have been associated with increased motivation to lose weight and greater patient weight loss success.[16,17]

Box 1
Key questions to ask regarding weight management in clinical practice

- Am I interested in counseling patients on diet, physical activity, and behavior change to lose weight?

- Have I had enough training where I feel comfortable and confident taking a lifestyle history and working collaboratively with patients to devise an evidence-based action plan?

- Do I have enough time available in my panel to accommodate frequent follow-up visits with patients every 2 to 4 weeks?

Box 2
5As counseling approach

- Assess
- Advise
- Agree
- Assist
- Arrange

Identifying Appropriate Patients for Weight Management—Assess

In order to identify appropriate patients for weight management, clinicians should determine the individual's degree of obesity, cardiovascular and other risk factors, and his or her readiness to change. This is the first step in the 5As approach, assess.

Obesity should be assessed by body mass index (BMI), which reflects an individual's degree of adiposity. BMI is typically an accurate approximation of adiposity, although this measure may be inaccurate for elite athletes with substantial muscle mass. BMI is often calculated automatically in electronic health records (**Box 3**). The US National Institutes of Health have classified BMI into 6 categories based upon the values-associated risks of death, diabetes, hypertension, and atherosclerotic coronary heart disease (**Table 1**). All classes of obesity are linked with high cardiovascular disease risk (BMI ≥30 kg/m^2) and should be target for weight management.[7] For patients with overweight, all may be eligible for weight management services; however, those patients who have other risk factors should be particularly targeted.

If the patient meets criteria for weight management based on BMI and risk factors, then the clinician and patient should agree that weight loss is appropriate. Clinicians should assess whether the patient is ready to make the changes necessary to succeed at losing weight.[7] If a patient does not currently have time available to dedicate to lifestyle, or if other issues are greater competing priorities, then deferring weight loss for another time is appropriate.

Educating About Health Risks and Benefits of Change—Advise

The second step in the 5As approach is advise, which gives the clinician the opportunity to educate the patient about his or her weight and the health risks linked with overweight and obesity. At minimum, patients should be advised that the greater the BMI, the greater the risk of cardiovascular disease, type 2 diabetes, and death.[7] Weight loss can reduce blood pressure, improve cholesterol profile and blood sugar, and decrease risk of developing diabetes. However, clinicians should be aware that weight loss through lifestyle changes has not led to decreased cardiovascular events.[18]

Box 3
Formula to calculate body mass index

$$BMI = \frac{Weight(kg)}{Height\ squared(m^2)}$$

Table 1
Classifications of body mass index

Category	BMI (kg/m²)	Eligible for Weight Management?
Underweight	<18.5	No
Normal weight	18.5–24.9	No
Overweight	25.0–29.9	Yes, particularly if risk factors: • Increased waist circumference (men >102 cm; women >88 cm) • Hypertension, type 2 diabetes mellitus, coronary heart disease, or other conditions associated with overweight/obesity
Class I obesity	30.0–34.9	Yes
Class II obesity	35.0–39.9	Yes
Class III obesity	≥40.0	Yes

Overweight and obesity have been linked to certain gastroenterological conditions such as gastroesophageal reflux disease (GERD) and nonalcoholic fatty liver disease (NAFLD).[1–20] Weight loss has been shown to improve these conditions.[21,22] Other gastroenterological conditions linked with obesity are described in other articles in this issue.

Collaborating to Establish Weight Management Goals—Agree

The third step in the 5As process is agree, in which the patient and clinician agree upon goals.[14,15] It is critical for clinicians to help their patients set goals that are quantifiable, achievable, and likely to lead to meaningful health benefits (eg, a goal of losing 5% of an individual's starting weight over the next 6 months to lower blood sugar and prevent the development of diabetes). The 2013 AHA/ACC/TOS guidelines suggest appropriate goals and health benefits that can be expected with certain weight losses (**Box 4**).[7]

Determining the Weight Management Strategy—Assist

The fourth step in the 5As process is Assist—in which the clinician and patient determine what weight management strategy will be pursed. In the following section, practice-based weight loss counseling is outlined briefly, and evidence regarding weight management programs is covered in more detail as most clinicians opt to refer patients to programs given their limited time and training in this area.

Box 4
Appropriate weight loss goals and associated health benefits

- Initial goal – 3% to 5% weight loss from starting weight over 3 to 6 months
  - Improves glucose, hemoglobin A1c, and triglycerides
  - Prevents development of type 2 diabetes mellitus in individuals with prediabetes
- Additional goal—5% to 10% weight loss from starting weight over 6 to 12 months
  - Improves blood pressure
  - Lowers low-density lipoprotein cholesterol and raises high-density lipoprotein cholesterol
  - Reduces need for medications

Practice-based weight loss counseling

For those clinicians who decide to take a leading role in weight management, the key duty involves engaging patients in a practice-based program that meets recommended guidelines. A systematic review found that behavioral interventions in clinical settings could result in weight losses of 3 kg over a 12-month period.[23] Clinicians should be aware that weight losses may be more modest when counseling occurs within typical clinical practice settings rather than the results achieved with more intensive weight loss programs.[24]

The clinician should assess weight and lifestyle histories, which can provide useful information about the origins of or maintaining factors for overweight and obesity, including success and difficulties with previous weight loss or maintenance efforts. Clinicians can consider having patients keep a food and activity journal for several days before their appointment to facilitate this process.

The 2013 AHA/ACC/TOS weight management guidelines suggest that clinicians' focus their counseling on a dietary strategy that results in moderately reduced caloric intake.[7] Patients can achieve this goal through a variety of strategies including:

- Limiting calories to 1200 to 1500 daily for women or 1500 to 1800 daily for men
- Prescribing a 500 to 750 calorie deficit from baseline calorie intake
- Following an evidence-based diet that promotes or restricts consumption of certain food types (low-fat diet, low-carbohydrate diet [eg, Atkins], very-low-fat vegetarian diet [eg, Ornish], high-fiber diet [eg, Volumetrics], or meal replacements)[7,25,26]

Dietary adherence has been associated with greater weight loss,[27] so engaging the patient in a discussion of all options and eliciting their preferences may be helpful. In addition to agreeing upon a specific dietary intervention, patients should be encouraged to pair the strategy with an appropriate behavioral intervention such as tracking calories or keeping a food diary to reinforce and support the behavior change.

Although physical activity has many health benefits and is critical for weight loss maintenance, clinicians avoid using increased physical activity as the sole weight loss strategy, as patients are unlikely to be successful losing weight. At 6 months, individuals who engage in physical activity alone lose about 2 kg of weight as compared to the 9 kg lost by those who changed their diet.[28] Increased physical activity can be an adjunct to dietary changes, but should not be the sole method for weight loss.

Referral to weight management services

For clinicians who prefer a more passive role in weight management, the key duties involve referring these individuals to evidence-based weight management programs and following up on patients' outcomes with these programs. The 2013 AHA/ACC/TOS guidelines recommend that clinicians refer patients to a high-intensity comprehensive lifestyle program for at least 6 months.[7] Programs should promote a lower-calorie diet and increased physical activity by using behavioral strategies. A high-intensity program should encourage individuals to attend at least 14 sessions over this 6-month period. Although scientific evidence supports the efficacy of such programs, clinicians should be aware that patients may have difficulties identifying programs in the community that meet these guidelines. For example, 1 study found that only 19% of programs in the community had high concordance with these guidelines, and relying only on information from the Internet is unlikely to yield results.[29] Clinicians who plan to rely on locally available weight management services should consider investing some time identifying and vetting programs to ensure that they are referring patients to evidence-based programs.

Alternatively, clinicians can consider referring patients to a center taking part in the US National Diabetes Prevention Program. The Diabetes Prevention Program (DPP) was a landmark trial that demonstrated how an intensive program of lifestyle changes and weight loss can delay the development of type 2 diabetes.[4,5] In March 2016, the US Centers for Medicare and Medicaid Services announced that Medicare will now provide these services as a covered benefit for beneficiaries at risk for type 2 diabetes.[30] The US Centers for Disease Control and Prevention (CDC) has established the US National Diabetes Prevention Program, which has set standards and guidelines for organizations to deliver CDC-recognized DPP programs in the community.[31] The DPP has also been offered through the YMCA through the YMCA of the USA Diabetes Prevention Program. Clinicians can now find CDC-recognized DPP programs in their communities online, which may facilitate referrals to this evidence-based program.

In addition, clinicians may also consider referring patients to commercial weight-loss programs. The 2013 AHA/ACC/TOS guidelines suggest that clinicians can consider referring patients to commercial programs that have evidence to support their efficacy.[7] Some commercial programs contain all components recommended by the 2013 AHA/ACC/TOS guidelines—high intensity, lower-calorie diet, increased physical activity, behavioral strategies, and support—while others do not (**Table 2**).

Clinicians considering referral to commercial programs might prioritize commercial programs that have all recommended components. However, not all commercial programs have been rigorously tested in long-term randomized controlled trials that report weight losses at 12 months or beyond.[26]

Currently, only 2 commercial weight loss programs—Weight Watchers and Jenny Craig—contain all components recommend in the 2013 AHA/ACC/TOS guidelines and consistently demonstrate their weight loss efficacy at 12 months in multiple randomized controlled trials (**Box 5**).[26] Weight Watchers participants monitor their food intake by tracking points and participate in group, one-on-one, or online support, while Jenny Craig participants use meal replacements and participate in one-on-one counseling. Both programs promote increased physical activity and use behavioral strategies such as self-monitoring and goal setting. The costs between the 2 programs differ substantially, although clinicians should be aware that the price of Jenny Craig

Table 2
Components of commercial weight loss programs

Program	High Intensity	Diet	Physical Activity	Behavior Strategies	Support
Weight Watchers	X	X	X	X	X
Jenny Craig	X	X	X	X	X
Nutrisystem	X	X	X	X	X
Curves	X	X	X	X	X
Health Management Resources (HMR)	X	X	X	X	X
Medifast	X	X	X	X	X
OPTIFAST	X	X	X	X	X
SlimFast	—	X	—	X	X
Atkins	—	X	X	X	X
The Biggest Loser Club	—	X	X	X	X
eDiets	—	X	X	—	X
Lose It!	—	X	X	X	X

Box 5
Weight loss results among weight Watchers' and Jenny Craig participants at 12 months

- Weight Watchers
  - Lost 3.5 to 4.3 kg at 12 months—at least 2.6% greater loss than control
- Jenny Craig
  - Lost 6.6 to 10.1 kg at 12 months—at least 4.9% greater loss than comparator

---

includes food for the month, whereas Weight Watchers prices do not. Weight Watchers has been suggested as the more cost-effective option.[32]

Monitoring Weight Loss Progress—Arrange

The final step in the 5As is—arrange, to set up follow-up with patients. In particular, arrange is often forgotten by clinicians, yet is a component associated with successful dietary change and weight loss.[17] This step enables clinicians to provide accountability for patients, cheerlead their successes, and maintain the long-term trusting relationship despite weight loss outcome.[11] Following up with patients to assess their progress within 3 months of the initial visit is appropriate for most patients, and a second follow-up is recommended at 6 months. These visits also provide an opportunity for the clinician to adjust medications in response to weight loss success. For example, many patients will need the dose of their antihypertensive medications lowered when they reach a 5% weight loss or beyond.

WEIGHT LOSS MAINTENANCE

Although patients can struggle to lose weight, maintaining weight loss can be more difficult. Observational studies have shown that about 20% of people can achieve and maintain a clinically significant weight loss for at least 1 year. Data from the US National Weight Control Registry indicates that successful strategies for weight maintenance include: high levels of physical activity (average 60 min/d), eating a low-calorie diet, self-monitoring weight, and maintaining a consistent eating pattern across the entire week.[33] In addition, randomized controlled trials have shown that monthly in-person contact leads to greater weight maintenance success than Web-based or self-directed efforts.[34,35] Therefore, ongoing support and monitoring by the clinician are likely needed for long-term success.

SUMMARY

Given the prevalence of overweight and obesity and their associated health conditions, clinicians will be increasingly tasked with the responsibility of addressing overweight and obesity. Clinicians can use the 5As approach—assess, advise, agree, assist, arrange—to facilitate weight management with their patients, regardless of whether the clinician prefers a leading or passive role in management. Given the limited time available and often insufficient training in obesity counseling, clinicians are likely to take a more passive role and refer patients to available services that should include any evidence-based local programs as well as CDC-recognized centers for the US National Diabetes Prevention Program and commercial weight-loss programs like Weight Watchers and Jenny Craig. Clinicians should continue to monitor patients' weight after a successful loss given high rates of weight regain.

REFERENCES

1. Ogden CL, Carroll MD, Kit BK, et al. Prevalence of childhood and adult obesity in the United States, 2011–2012. JAMA 2014;311:806–14.
2. Flegal KM, Graubard BI, Williamson DF, et al. Cause-specific excess deaths associated with underweight, overweight, and obesity. JAMA 2007;298:2028–37.
3. Appel LJ, Champagne CM, Harsha DW, et al, Writing Group of the PREMIER Collaborative Research Group. Effects of comprehensive lifestyle modification on blood pressure control: main results of the PREMIER clinical trial. JAMA 2003;289:2083–93.
4. Knowler WC, Barrett-Connor E, Fowler SE, et al. Reduction in the incidence of type 2 diabetes with lifestyle intervention or metformin. N Engl J Med 2002;346: 393–403.
5. Knowler WC, Fowler SE, Hamman RF, et al, Diabetes Prevention Program Research Group. 10-year follow-up of diabetes incidence and weight loss in the Diabetes Prevention Program Outcomes Study. Lancet 2009;374:1677–86.
6. U.S. Preventive Services Task Force. Obesity in adults: screening and management. Rockville (MD): U.S. Preventive Services Task Force; 2012. Available at: http://www.uspreventiveservicestaskforce.org/Page/Document/UpdateSummaryFinal/obesity-in-adults-screening-and-management. Accessed May 17, 2016.
7. Jensen MD, Ryan DH, Apovian CM, et al. 2013 AHA/ACC/TOS guideline for the management of overweight and obesity in adults: a report of the American College of Cardiology/American Heart Association Task Force on Practice Guidelines and The Obesity Society. Circulation 2014;129:S102–38.
8. Kushner RF. Barriers to providing nutrition counseling by physicians: a survey of primary care practitioners. Prev Med 1995;24:546–52.
9. Bleich SN, Bennett WL, Gudzune KA, et al. National survey of US primary care physicians' perspectives about causes of obesity and solutions to improve care. BMJ Open 2012;2(6).
10. Gudzune KA, Clark JM, Appel LJ, et al. Primary care providers' communication with patients during weight counseling: a focus group study. Patient Educ Couns 2012;89:152–7.
11. Bennett WL, Gudzune KA, Appel LJ, et al. Insights from the POWER practice-based weight loss trial: a focus group study on the PCP's role in weight management. J Gen Intern Med 2014;29:50–8.
12. Bennett WL, Wang NY, Gudzune KA, et al. Satisfaction with primary care provider involvement is associated with greater weight loss: results from the practice-based POWER trial. Patient Educ Couns 2015;98:1099–105.
13. Gudzune KA, Bennett WL, Cooper LA, et al. Perceived judgment about weight can negatively influence weight loss: a cross-sectional study of overweight and obese patients. Prev Med 2014;62:103–7.
14. Whitlock EP, Orleans CT, Pender N, et al. Evaluating primary care behavioral counseling interventions: an evidence-based approach. Am J Prev Med 2002; 22:267–84.
15. Serdula MK, Khan LK, Dietz WH. Weight loss counseling revisited. JAMA 2003; 289:1747–50.
16. Jay M, Gillespie C, Schlair S, et al. Physicians' use of the 5As in counseling obese patients: is the quality of counseling associated with patients' motivation and intention to lose weight? BMC Health Serv Res 2010;10:159.
17. Alexander SC, Cox ME, Boling Turner CL, et al. Do the five A's work when physicians counsel about weight loss? Fam Med 2011;43:179–84.

18. Look AHEAD Research Group. Cardiovascular effects of intensive lifestyle intervention in type 2 diabetes. N Engl J Med 2013;369:145–54.
19. Hampel H, Abraham NS, El-Seraq HB. Meta-analysis: obesity and the risk for gastroesophageal reflux disease and its complications. Ann Intern Med 2005; 143:199–211.
20. Clark JM. The epidemiology of nonalcoholic fatty liver disease in adults. J Clin Gastroenterol 2006;40(Suppl 1):S5–10.
21. Kaltenbach T, Crockett S, Gerson LB. Are lifestyle measures effective in patients with gastroesophageal reflux disease? An evidence-based approach. Arch Intern Med 2006;166:965–71.
22. Clark JM. Weight loss as a treatment for nonalcoholic fatty liver disease. J Clin Gastroenterol 2006;40(Suppl 1):S39–43.
23. LeBlanc ES, O'Conner E, Whitlock EP, et al. Effectiveness of primary care – relevant treatments for obesity in adults: a systematic evidence review for the U.S. Preventive Services task force. Ann Intern Med 2011;155:434–47.
24. Jolly K, Lewis A, Beach J, et al. Comparison of range of commercial or primary care led weight reduction programmes with minimal intervention control for weight loss in obesity: Lighten UP randomised controlled trial. BMJ 2011;343: d6500.
25. Johnston BC, Kanters S, Bandayrel K, et al. Comparison of weight loss among named diet programs in overweight and obese adults: a meta-analysis. JAMA 2014;312:923–33.
26. Gudzune KA, Doshi RS, Mehta AK, et al. Efficacy of commercial weight-loss programs: an updated systematic review. Ann Intern Med 2015;162:501–12.
27. Dansinger ML, Gleason JA, Griffith JL, et al. Comparison of the Atkins, Ornish, Weight Watchers, and Zone diets for weight loss and heart disease risk reduction: a randomized trial. JAMA 2005;293:43–53.
28. Wing RR, Venditti E, Jakicic JM, et al. Lifestyle intervention in overweight individuals with a family history of diabetes. Diabetes Care 1998;21:350–9.
29. Bloom B, Mehta AK, Clark JM, et al. Guideline-concordant weight-loss programs in an urban area are uncommon and difficult to identify through the Internet. Obesity (Silver Spring) 2016;24:583–8.
30. Department of Health and Human Services. Certification of Medicare Diabetes Prevention Program. 2016. Available at: https://www.cms.gov/Research-Statistics-Data-and-Systems/Research/ActuarialStudies/Downloads/Diabetes-Prevention-Certification-2016-03-14.pdf. Accessed May 17, 2016.
31. Centers for Disease Control and Prevention. National Diabetes Prevention Program. 2016. Available at: http://www.cdc.gov/diabetes/prevention/index.html. Accessed May 17, 2016.
32. Finkelstein EA, Kruger E. Meta- and cost-effectiveness analysis of commercial weight loss strategies. Obesity (Silver Spring) 2014;22:1942–51.
33. Wing RR, Phelan S. Long-term weight loss maintenance. Am J Clin Nutr 2005;82: 222S–5S.
34. Wing RR, Tate DF, Gorin AA, et al. A Self-Regulation Program for Maintenance of Weight Loss. N Engl J Med 2006;355:1563–71.
35. Svetkey LP, Stevens VJ, Brantley PJ, et al. Comparison of strategies for sustaining weight loss: the weight loss maintenance randomized controlled trial. JAMA 2008;299:1139–48.

Pharmacotherapy in Treatment of Obesity

Jeanette N. Keith, MD[a,b,c]

KEYWORDS

- Pharmacotherapy • Colon cancer • Hepatitis C • Nonalcoholic fatty liver disease
- Brain-gut axis

KEY POINTS

- The gut-brain axis is a major pathway in energy metabolism and is targeted by antiobesity medications to facilitate short- and long-term weight loss.
- The use of antiobesity medication is an important adjunctive intervention in the treatment of morbid obesity.
- Medical weight management that includes pharmacologic interventions improves weight loss outcomes and clinical outcomes in the management of chronic gastrointestinal conditions including hepatitis C, nonalcoholic fatty liver disease, and colon cancer.

INTRODUCTION

Common disease states in gastroenterology are more effectively treated in an obese patient when weight loss is incorporated into the treatment plan. Strategies that seek to achieve weight loss improve outcomes in the treatment of hepatitis C, nonalcoholic fatty liver disease, and colorectal cancer.[1–3] In the management of hepatitis C, obesity is a pretreatment predictor of response and is associated with a lower response to antiviral therapy.[4] Weight reduction also reduces the risk and improves outcomes for colon cancer development.[5] Medical weight management using only dietary modification and behavioral changes as primary methods for the treatment of obesity has been limited by a high recidivism rate and weight regain.[6] Pharmacologic therapy is an important adjunctive intervention that improves short- and long-term outcomes in the management of obese patients.[7,8] Unfortunately, many of the earlier medications approved for clinical use have been associated with adverse events and complications leading to their withdrawal from the US market.[9] However, the recent development of highly effective pharmacotherapy with fewer side effects has generated a renewed interest in medical weight management.[10] This article reviews currently available drug therapy with a focus on pharmacotherapy-approved long-term weight management in obese

Disclosure: Speaker Bureau, National Dairy Council, Inc.
[a] Alabama College of Osteopathic Medicine, Dothan, AL, USA; [b] Decatur Morgan Hospital, Department of Medicine, Section of Gastroenterology, Decatur, AL, USA; [c] Decatur Gastroenterology Associates, P.C., 1103 15th Avenue Southeast, Decatur, AL 35601, USA
E-mail address: mygastrodoc@bhip.us.com

Gastroenterol Clin N Am 45 (2016) 663–672
http://dx.doi.org/10.1016/j.gtc.2016.07.011
0889-8553/16/© 2016 Elsevier Inc. All rights reserved.

individuals without diabetes since 2012, encouraging the use of these tools in the practice of gastroenterology. As the understanding of the pathways that regulate food intake and energy expenditure increase, new drug therapies will emerge and expand the number of available tools. Certain noradrenergic sympathomimetic drugs (benzphatamine, phendimetrazine) that have been approved for short-term use are excluded from this discussion because the general use of sympathomimetic drugs for long-term weight loss is discouraged. Phentermine and tenuate are the notable exceptions.[11]

DRUG TARGETS

Obesity occurs when there is an imbalance between energy intake and energy expenditure.[7,12] There are peripheral and central signals as well as hormonal and neural pathways that regulate food intake and body fat mass. Although a detailed discussion is beyond the scope of this article, clinicians should have a basic understanding of these mechanisms because the signals regulate when an individual eats, how much they eat, and when they achieve satiety. Furthermore, following intentional weight loss, these signals result in adaptations that stimulate hunger, increase food intake, reduce the metabolic rate, and predispose to weight regain. These influences directly impact the management of gastrointestinal (GI) diseases and general medical weight management.[13] **Figs. 1** and **2** summarize the interactions between the central and

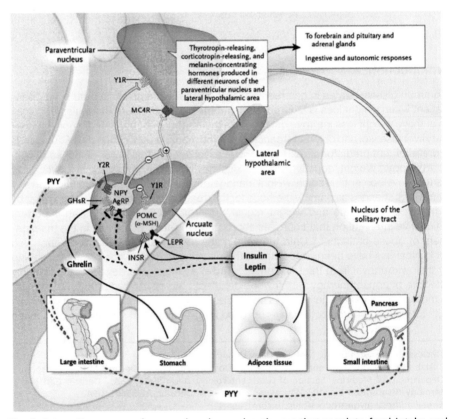

Fig. 1. Interactions among hormonal and neural pathways that regulate food intake and body fat mass. (*From* Korner J, Liebel RL. To eat or not to eat: how the gut talks to the brain. N Engl J Med 2003;349:927; with permission.)

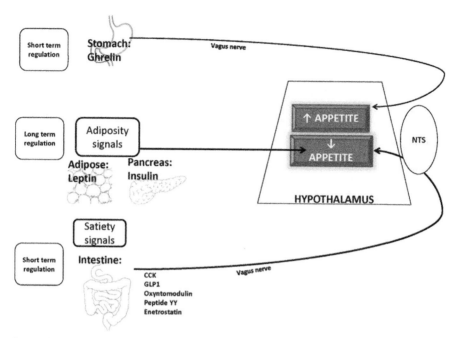

Fig. 2. Short- and long-term regulators of energy intake. CCK, cholecystokinin; NTS, nucleus tractus solitaries. (*Adapted from* Misra M. Obesity pharmacotherapy: current perspectives and future directions. Curr Cardiol Rev 2013;9:35; with permission.)

peripheral pathways that regulate food intake.[14] Food intake is driven by the sum of the signals as opposed to an individual signal. There is also redundancy in the pathways such that alternate paths can override or bypass signals from the primary pathways. Leptin, derived from the adipose tissue, and insulin from the pancreas are the main long-term signals and act at the level of the arcuate nucleus in the brain.[15] They also modulate the peripheral short-term signals that regulate food intake. In the arcuate nucleus, leptin and ghrelin interface with two major populations of neurons that result in either increased food intake or reduced food intake. The neurons that promote food intake express agouti-related peptide and neuropeptide Y. The other neurons that inhibit food intake express pro-opiomelanocortin (POMC) and cocaine- and amphetamine-regulated transcript. In addition to signals from leptin and ghrelin, these neurons are regulated by short-term signals from the periphery including glucose, insulin, glucagon-like peptide (GLP)-1, peptide YY, and oxyntomodulin. Of physiologic and clinical significance, neurotransmitters (dopamine, serotonin, γ-aminobutyric acid [GABA], and norepinephrine) from other parts of the brain impact and regulate the POMC neuronal activity.[16]

The short-term signals of energy intake and metabolism originate from the stomach and intestines.[16–18] The stomach produces the hormone ghrelin, which stimulates hunger before a meal. It is the only orexigenic signal in the periphery. There are also mechanoreceptors on the stomach wall that signal fullness and satiety following a meal via vagal afferent neurons. The vagus nerve is involved in nutrient sensing along the length of the GI tract. It provides information to the brain regarding digestibility, pH, and perceptions of taste, and detects changes in leptin and ghrelin levels. In the proximal intestine, intraluminal nutrients (ie, protein and fat) stimulate the release of cholecystokinin from intestinal I cells, which suppresses hunger when it is transmitted centrally via the vagus nerve. There are specialized enteroendocrine cells called L cells in the gut that produce a metabolically active peptide, peptide YY, which slows intestinal motility resulting in increased satiety and is the so-called "ileal brake." Another regulatory signal comes from incretins that are gut-derived peptide hormones that increase insulin release from the pancreas and inhibit glucagon release from the pancreas. These signals are released into circulation in proportion to the calories ingested. The net result is a lowering of the blood glucose level and modulation of the insulin signal. Incretins also slow gastric emptying and may directly reduce food intake. They are involved in vagal and central nervous system effects related to appetite regulation. The two most studied incretins are GLP-1 and glucose-dependent insulinotrophic polypeptide. They are inactivated by the enzyme dipeptidyl peptidase-4. Understanding the role of incretins in glucose homeostasis and their effect on insulin has led to the development of new drug therapies (eg, Liraglutide) used in the treatment of diabetes. Other incretins are pancreatic polypeptide, oxyntomodulin, and amylin, which will serve as future drug targets in the management of diabetes and obesity in patients without diabetes. Of interest, gut organisms or microbiota can activate the vagus nerve and may directly influence energy homeostasis. These gut organisms are thought to cause a low-grade inflammatory state that alters the signaling in the gut and contribute to the development of obesity and other conditions, such as inflammatory bowel syndrome. Hence, the emergence of prebiotics and probiotics to treat such clinical conditions.

Current antiobesity drug targets are designed to disrupt the gut-brain axis.[19] Most agents are focused on disrupting mechanisms that control appetite and are designed to stimulate the POMC neurons promoting satiety with small food intake. The net result is less food intake and increased weight loss, particularly when there is a simultaneous increase in energy expenditure. The exception is the pancreatic and gastric lipase inhibitor, orlistat, which decreases the absorption of fat calories promoting weight loss by a reduction in caloric intake.

DRUG THERAPY
Diethylpropion

One of the oldest drugs available is diethylpropion (Tenuate), which was approved in the 1960s for short-term use (ie, 3 months) in weight management, at a dose of 75 mg po TID, one hour before meals.[20] It is a norepinephrine-releasing agent that typically results in a 3.0-kg weight loss above diet alone. Its use is limited by side effects including cardiac (palpitations, elevated blood pressure, ischemic events), GI (dry mouth, constipation, diarrhea), and central nervous system (anxiety, overstimulation, insomnia, dysphoria, psychosis) to name a few. Contraindications include anxiety disorders, uncontrolled hypertension, seizures, cardiac disease, hyperthyroidism, the use of monoamine oxidase inhibitors (MOAI), glaucoma, and a history of drug abuse. As with all obesity medications, use during pregnancy and breastfeeding is contraindicated.

Phentermine

Phentermine is also a norepinephrine-releasing agent similar to dietylpropion.[21] It was also released in the 1960s for short-term use of 3 months for weight management but was withdrawn from the market because of the emergence of valvular heat disease when used in combination with fenfluramine, a serotonin 5-HT$_{2B}$ receptor agonist that functioned as a serotonin reuptake inhibitor. The use of the medication and duration of therapy has been debated since the phentermine-fenfluramine ("phen-fen") combination was withdrawn from the market but it has been safely used as a single agent for up to 1 year. As a single agent, it produces an average weight loss of 3.6 kg above diet and lifestyle changes alone. It is marketed as Adipex in 15- to 37.5-mg capsules and 37.5-mg tablets. There is a dispersible oral tablet, Suprenza, available in 15-, 30-, and 37.5-mg strengths. The side effect profile and contraindications are the same as dietylpropion given the same mechanism of action. Pregnancy and breastfeeding are contraindications.

Orlistat

Orlistat (Xenical or Alli) is a pancreatic and gastric lipase inhibitor.[22] It prevents the absorption of approximately 30% of the fat calories in the diet, resulting in a net reduction of total calories metabolized. It was approved in 1999 as one of the first drugs for long-term medical weight management. The net weight loss above dietary management is 2.9 to 3.4 kg with mean weight loss of 2.9% to 3.4% at 1 year, at doses of 60-120 mg TID. Orlistat is associated with decreased absorption of the fat-soluble vitamins, steatorrhea, oily spotting, increased flatulence, fecal urgency, increased defecation, and fecal incontinence. In 2010, there was a black box warning added because of the occurrence of severe liver injury that had been reported rarely with use of this medication. There is also a risk of increased urinary oxalate excretion leading to oxalate nephrolithiasis and oxalate nephropathy with renal failure in some patients. During orlistat administration, the addition of a multivitamin daily but temporally separated from the orlistat dose by at least 2 hours is recommended. Contraindications include cyclosporine use, chronic malabsorption, and cholestasis. Patients taking warfarin, levothyroxine, antiepileptic drugs, paricalcitol, vitamin D analogues, and amiodarone are encouraged to avoid use of this medication. Pregnancy and breastfeeding are contraindications.

Lorcaserin

Locaserin (Belviq) is a serotonin 5-HT_{2c} receptor agonist that is an anorexiant.[23] Approved in 2012 for use in chronic weight management, it may be used in obese patients with diabetes, hypertension, and/or dyslipidemia and the general obese patient. It produces weight reduction of 3.6 kg above diet alone and a 3.6% weight reduction at 1 year, at a maximal dose of 20 mg per day in 1-2 divided doses. Because the drug has a greater affinity for the serotonin 5-HT_{2c} receptor as opposed to the serotonin 5-HT_{2B} receptor (eg, fenfluramine) at therapeutic doses, the risk of valvular heart disease is thought to be low. To minimize risk of an adverse event, locaserin should be discontinued if patients do not lose 5% of the starting body weight in 12 weeks. Side effects include headache, nausea, dry mouth, fatigue, dizziness, and constipation. This medication should be used with extreme caution in patients taking selective serotonin reuptake inhibitors, serotonin and norepinephrine reuptake inhibitor/MOAI, triptans, St. John's wort, bupropion, and dextromethorphan. Because there are multiple drug interactions, use of a drug reference or consultation with a pharmacist may be indicated. Pregnancy and breastfeeding are contraindications.

Phentermine/Topiramate

Topiramate is a GABA receptor modulator.[24,25] GABA is an inhibitory neurotransmitter in the central nervous system that reduces food intake beyond the effects of the POMC and cocaine- and amphetamine-regulated transcript receptors. Topiramate is thought to reduce food intake by a variety of steps including augmentation of GABA activity. The result is appetite suppression and satiety enhancement. However, because of side effects at a therapeutic dose when used as a single agent, it is not indicated as monotherapy for weight management. At a lower dose in combination with phentermine, topiramate is approved for medical weight management. The fixed drug combination is marketed as Qsymia. The starting dose is 3.75 mg of phentermine and 23 mg of topiramate administered daily for 2 weeks. The recommended daily dose is increased to 7.5 mg of phentermine and 46 mg of topiramate. Although seldom done, the dose can be adjusted to the high-dose regimen of 15 mg of phentermine and 92 mg of topiramate if weight loss is inadequate. The weight loss with standard dosing is 6.6 kg and with the higher dosing is 8.6 kg above diet alone. The weight loss at 1 year for the standard dose and the high dose are 6.6% and 8.6%, respectively. The most common side effects reported are insomnia, dry mouth, constipation, dizziness, and dysguesia. Other side effects include adverse reactions from each of the components as noted with phentermine and topiramate components. Birth defects have been reported because of the use of this fixed-dose combination therapy.[25] It is best to avoid use in pregnant women, those who are planning pregnancy, and those of child-bearing age. If the use of the medication is indicated in this high-risk population, contraception is encouraged. Women who become pregnant while using phentermine/topiramate are asked to enroll themselves in the AED Pregnancy Registry (1-888-233-2334). Additional information is available at www.aedpregnancyregistry.org. Additional contraindications to therapy are breastfeeding, hyperthyroidism, concurrent therapy with MOAI, and the use of sympathomimetic amines. Of interest, Qsymia is not available worldwide. The European Medicine Agency rejected its application for approval citing its adverse reactions and potential long-term effects.

Naltrexone/Bupropion

The fixed-dose combination of naltrexone-bupropion (Contrave) is administered in an increasing stair-step fashion.[26] During Week 1, one tablet with 8 mg naltrexone and 90 mg of bupropion is given once a day. During the second week, the dose is increased to one tablet twice a day. In Week 3, two tablets are taken in the morning and one at night. By Week 4, the dose is increased to two tablets orally twice a day. At maximal therapy (32 mg of naltrexone and 390 mg of bupropion), the expected weight loss is 4.8% at 1 year. If patients have not lost 5% of their starting weight by 12 weeks, the medication should be discontinued. Because the combination drug causes moderate delay in gastric emptying, nausea with vomiting is a common side effect. Individuals may also experience constipation, headache, insomnia, and dry mouth. There may be a transient rise in blood pressure (1–2 mm Hg) and increased heart rate during the first 12 weeks of therapy. The use of this combination therapy is contraindicated in patients with uncontrolled hypertension, seizure disorders, eating disorders, drug or alcohol withdrawal, and those using MOAI, and during pregnancy and breastfeeding.

Liraglutide

Liraglutide is a GLP-1 agonist marketed under the brand name Saxenda.[27] Although it is primarily used in the management of type 2 diabetes, it was approved for chronic weight management in 2014. Unlike the other therapies for medical weight management that are available in capsule or pill form, liraglutide is administered by subcutaneous injection once a day. However, it is generally well tolerated. The initial dose is 0.6 mg subcutaneously daily for 1 week. The dose is then increased weekly by 0.6-mg doses to the target dose of 3 mg daily. The typical weight loss is 5.8% at 1 year. Regular monitoring on this therapy is required. In 34% of patients, there is an increase in heart rate greater than 10 beats per minute. In 5%, the resting heart rate increases greater than 20 beats per minute, and in 6% there is a resting tachycardia greater than 100 beats per minute. The medication should be stopped if there is a sustained tachycardia. If a weight loss of 4% has not occurred by Week 16, the medication should be stopped. If one experiences an adverse reaction at the higher dose, the medication should be stopped because weight loss at the lower levels has not been established. Limitations to its use include injection site reaction, nausea, vomiting, pancreatitis, constipation, diarrhea, gallbladder disease, increased resting heart rate, suicidal behavior, worsening depression, unusual changes in mood or behavior, and hypoglycemia when taken in combination with other medications for diabetes. Of note, in rats and mice, liraglutide has been shown to cause thyroid cancer. Therefore, if the patient or their family members have or have had medullary thyroid cancer or multiple endocrine neoplasia type 2, the drug should not be used. The use of a different antiobesity medication should be considered if there is a history of suicidal thoughts or actions.

PATIENT ASSESSMENT

To enhance the success of medical weight management within the gastroenterology practice, there should be structure within the practice to assess the patient's candidacy for drug therapy before treatment, identify potential contraindications for the specific drug therapies, initiate treatment, provide continual monitoring, and provide general support during active treatment.[28] To simplify the process, a 24-hour dietary recall and food logs can be used to assess compliance with dietary modification. During the initial clinic visit, it is important to obtain a measured height and an actual weight on the same scale that will be used during follow-up visits. Waist circumference should also be measured and the body mass index calculated to determine the obesity-associated risks. Changes in body weight, waist circumference, body mass index, and a record of their physical activity can serve as verification of compliance with dietary and lifestyle modification.

Once the decision is made to begin pharmacologic therapy, the patient should be assessed at baseline, monthly for 3 months, and then every 3 months thereafter in the absence of an adverse event. We record the vitals with attention to blood pressure and pulse, a measured weight, and the waist circumference. Their log of calories and physical activity is reviewed each visit. If the weight loss targets are met and there are no adverse events, the medications are continued. If there is an adverse event or failure to lose weight, a different agent or surgical intervention is considered. One may also consider antiobesity devices for additional weight loss.

DEFINING SUCCESS

Antiobesity medications are not a perfect solution to the obesity epidemic. Effective weight loss requires dietary modification and regular increased physical activity in combination with pharmacotherapy when clinically indicated.[29] In our practice, all patients are given a trial of diet and exercise under our supervision to confirm that they are making the necessary foundational lifestyle changes over a 3- to 6-month period. Antiobesity medications are used when there is an inability to lose weight with diet alone, when maintenance of successful weight loss is compromised, and when weight regain occurs. It is appropriate to consider drug use in postbypass patients who are struggling or have achieved the maximal weight loss benefits of surgery alone.

Historically, success in medical weight management was defined as weight loss to the ideal body weight. However, few individuals were successful in reaching this goal, even after bariatric surgery.[30] In contrast, weight loss of 5% to 10% of total body weight has been shown to have a significant impact on cardiovascular and metabolic parameters.[31] Intentional weight loss of 5% to 10% is associated with a more than 9% reduction in colon cancer[32] and a 15% reduction in all-cause mortality.[33] Based on these data, realistic and achievable goals for weight loss from nonsurgical methods have been determined. The current definition of success in medical weight management is more appropriately defined as achieving the physiologically important weight loss of 5% to 10% body weight and achieving risk reduction relative to obesity-related comorbidities.[34] When pharmacotherapy is used in conjunction with dietary and behavior modification, drug therapy enhances weight loss and improves long-term weight maintenance.[8] Beginning in 2012, the Food and Drug Administration released several new drug therapies to assist in the management of obesity. The new drugs were evaluated using robust criteria and must result in a minimum of 5% weight reduction for their initial approval. When antiobesity medications are combined with diet and behavioral changes, a greater percentage of individuals achieve the metabolically significant 5% to 10% weight loss. This should translate into a 1 lb per week weight loss or 2 kg loss in the first month. There should be a 5% weight loss in the first 3 to 6 months and maintenance of at least 5% long-term. When drugs are used in addition to diet, exercise, and lifestyle changes, weight loss of 10% to 15% is a very good response and greater than 15% is considered excellent.[35] There is no information regarding continuous drug treatment beyond 4 years. Clinical judgment and incorporation of emerging science into clinical practice are indicated regarding long-term treatment duration. Medical noncompliance, active drug or excessive alcohol use, and pregnancy should be absolute indications to discontinue the use of medications and active weight reduction.

SUMMARY

The treatment of common GI disorders and responsiveness to disease-specific medications in such conditions as hepatitis C are improved in obese patients when medical weight management is included in their treatment strategies. Although diet and exercise alone have had limited success in the past, the addition of pharmacotherapy improves outcomes and is an important adjunctive treatment option in the treatment of obesity. With the redefinition of success in medical weight management, reaching the metabolic important weight loss of 5% to 10% is achievable for most patients. Preintervention assessment and routine reassessment are essential. Recognition of indications to discontinue therapy when clinical targets are not met is a new focus and key to preventing adverse outcomes. Understanding the pathways involved in energy intake and energy expenditure allows clinicians to identify potential therapeutic targets, effectively incorporate pharmacotherapy into their clinical practices, and monitor for potential adverse events.

REFERENCES

1. Charlton MR, Pockros PJ, Harrison SA. Impact of obesity on treatment of chronic hepatitis C. Hepatology 2006;43:1177–86.
2. Fabbrini E, Sullivan S, Klein S. Obesity and nonalcoholic fatty liver disease: biochemical, metabolic and clinical implications. Hepatology 2010;51:679–89.
3. Frezza EE, Wachtel MS. Chiriva-Internati. Influence of obesity on the risk of developing colon cancer. Gut 2006;55:285–91.
4. Negro F, Clement S. Impact of obesity, steatosis, and insulin resistance on progression and response to therapy of hepatitis C. J Viral Hepat 2009;16:681–8.
5. Aleksandrova K, Nimptsch K, Pischon T. Influence of obesity and related metabolic alterations on colorectal cancer risk. Curr Nutr Rep 2013;2:1–9.

6. Weiss EC, Galusk DA, Kettel KK, et al. Weight regain in U.S. adults who experienced substantial weight loss, 1999-2002. Am J Prev Med 2007;33:34–40.

7. Rodgers RJ, Tschop MH, Wilding JPH. Anti-obesity drugs: past, present and future. Dis Model Mech 2012;5:621–6.

8. Yanovski SZ, Yanovski JA. Long-term drug treatment for obesity: a systematic and clinical review. JAMA 2014;311:74–86.

9. Kang JG, Park C. Anti-obesity drugs: a review about their effects and safety. Diabetes Metab J 2012;36:13–25.

10. Kim GW, Lin JE, Blomain ES, et al. Antiobesity pharmacotherapy: new drugs and emerging targets. Clin Pharmacol Ther 2014;95:53–66.

11. Glandt M, Raz I. Present and future: pharmacologic treatment of obesity. J Obes 2011;2011:1–13.

12. Hill JO, Wyatt HR, Peters JC. Energy balance and obesity. Circulation 2012;126:126–32.

13. Dulloo AG, Montani JP. Pathways from dieting to weight regain, to obesity and to the metabolic syndrome: an overview. Obes Rev 2015;16(Suppl 1):1–6.

14. Korner J, Leibel RL. To eat or not to eat-how the gut talks to the brain. N Engl J Med 2003;349:926–8.

15. Misra M. Obesity pharmacotherapy: current perspectives and future directions. Curr Cardiol Rev 2013;9:33–54.

16. Jones BJ, Bloom SR. The new era of drug therapy for obesity: the evidence and expectations. Drugs 2015;75:935–45.

17. Hussain SS, Bloom SR. The regulation of food intake by the gut-brain axis: implications for obesity. Int J Obes 2013;37:625–33.

18. Konturek SJ, Konturek JW, Pawlik T, et al. Brain-gut axis and its role in the control of food intake. J Physiol Pharmacol 2004;55:137–54.

19. Chaudhri OB, Wynne K, Bloom SR. Can gut hormones control appetite and prevent obesity? Diabetes Care 2008;31:S284–9.

20. Apovian CM, Aronne LJ, Bessesen DH, et al. Pharmacologic management of obesity: an endocrine society clinical practice guideline. J Clin Endocrinol Metab 2015;100:342–62.

21. McMahon FG, Fujioka K, Singh BN, et al. Efficacy and safety of sibutramine in obese white and African American patients with hypertension: a 1 year, double-blind, placebo controlled, multicenter trial. Arch Intern Med 2000;160:2185–91.

22. Davidson MH, Hauptman J, DiGirolamo M, et al. Weight control and risk factor reduction in obese subjects treated for 2 years with orlistat: a randomized controlled trial. JAMA 1999;281:235–42.

23. Smith SR, Weissman NJ, Anderson CM, et al. Multicenter, placebo-controlled trial of locaserin for weight management. N Engl J Med 2010;363:245–56.

24. Gadde KM, Allison DB, Ryan DH, et al. Effects of low-dose, controlled-release, phentermine plus topiramate combination on weight and associated comorbidities in overweight and obese adults (CONQUER): a randomized, placebo-controlled, phase 3 trial. Lancet 2011;377:1341–52.

25. Available at: http://www.fda.gov/downloads/drugs/drugsafety/postmarketdrugsafteyinformationforpatientsandprovidera/UMC312598.pdf. Accessed June 1, 2016.

26. Wadden TA, Foreyt JP, Foster GD, et al. Weight loss with naltrexone SR/bupropion SR on weight and obesity-related risk factors (COR-II). Obesity (Silver Spring) 2011;19:110–20.

27. Pi-Sunyer X, Astrup A, Fujioka K, et al. A Randomized, controlled trial of 3.0 mg if Liraglutide in weight management. N Engl J Med 2015;373:11–22.

28. Bray GA, Ryan DH. Medical therapy for the patient with obesity. Circulation 2012; 125:1695–703.

29. Avenell A, Broom J, Brown TJ, et al. Systematic review of the long-term effects and economic consequences of treatments for obesity and implications for health improvement. Health Technol Assess 2004;8:iii–iv, 1–182.

30. Sumithran P, Proietto J. The defense of body weight: a physiological basis for weight regain after weight loss. Clin Sci (Lond) 2013;124:231–41.

31. Brown RE, Kuk JL. Consequences of obesity and weight loss: a devil's advocate position. Obes Rev 2015;16:77–87.

32. Parker ED, Folsom AR. Intentional weight loss and incidence of obesity-related cancers: the Iowa's Health study. Int J Obes 2003;27:1447–52.

33. Kritchevsky SB, Beavers KM, Miller ME, et al. Intentional weight loss an all-cause mortality: a meta-analysis of randomized clinical trials. PLoS One 2015;10: e0121993.

34. Kraschnewski JL, Boan J, Esposito J, et al. Long-term weight loss maintenance in the United States. Int J Obes 2010;34:1644–54.

35. Bray GA. Obesity in adults: overview of management. UptoDate 2015. Available at: www.uptodate.com. Accessed June 25, 2016.

Endoscopic Management

Michael C. Bennett, MD[a], Ricardo Badillo, MD[a],
Shelby Sullivan, MD[b],*

KEYWORDS

- Obesity • Endoscopic bariatric therapy • Intragastric balloon • Transpyloric shuttle
- Endoscopic sleeve gastroplasty • Primary obesity surgery endoluminal
- Aspiration therapy • Duodenal-jejunal bypass liner

KEY POINTS

- Multiple devices and procedures for primary treatment of obesity and treatment of weight regain after Roux-en-Y gastric bypass (RYGB) are now available.
- In many cases, efficacy of these procedures and devices has been demonstrated with randomized sham-controlled or nonsham-controlled trials.
- Multiple gastric and small bowel devices for weight loss are currently being evaluated or have US pivotal trials planned for US Food and Drug Administration approval.
- Endoscopic revision of the gastrojejunostomy for weight regain after RYGB is an effective treatment for weight regain as shown in a randomized sham-controlled trial for patients with dilation of the gastrojejunostomy.

INTRODUCTION

Endoscopic bariatric therapy (EBT) has the potential to play a significant part in both the primary and secondary therapy of obesity. EBT may have more effectiveness than lifestyle therapy alone or medications,[1] and while EBT generally is less effective than bariatric surgery, it has fewer complications and is less expensive. In 2015, the US Food and Drug Administration (FDA) approved 2 new endoscopic bariatric devices for primary obesity treatment: the ReShape Integrated Dual Balloon System (ReShape Dual Balloon, ReShape Medical, San Clemente, California) and the Orbera Intragastric Balloon System (Apollo Endosurgery, Austin, Texas). Several therapies are available for gastrojejunostomy revision for weight regain after Roux-en-Y gastric bypass (RYGB).

This article will discuss devices or techniques with FDA approval (including devices that have general FDA approval for nonspecific uses in the gastrointestinal [GI] tract),

Disclosures: Contracted Research for ReShape Medical, GI Dynamics, Aspire Bariatrics, USGI Medical, Obalon Therapeutics, BAROnova, Paion; consultant for USGI Medical, Obalon, Elilra Therapeutics (S. Sullivan). None (M.C. Bennett and R. Badillo).
[a] Division of Gastroenterology, Washington University School of Medicine, St Louis, MO, USA;
[b] Division of Gastroenterology, University of Colorado School of Medicine, Mail Stop B158, Academic Office 1, 12631 E. 17th Ave, Aurora, CO 80045, USA
* Corresponding author.
E-mail address: shelby.sullivan@ucdenver.edu

as well as those with currently running or planned US pivotal trials for FDA approval. EBT methods, their results and risks, are outlined.

PRIMARY THERAPY

The American Society for Gastrointestinal Endoscopy (ASGE) recently released a position statement supporting the use of EBT in conjunction with a multidisciplinary weight loss program for long-term obesity treatment.[2] EBT can be considered in those who have failed weight loss or maintenance with lifestyle intervention alone and meet BMI criteria for particular treatment modalities, or Have medical conditions that require weight loss for additional therapy (eg, bridge therapy to weight loss surgery). Current approved and investigational devices for primary EBT include space-occupying devices, tissue apposition devices, and nutrient-diverting devices.

Intragastric Balloons

The use of intragastric balloon (IGB) therapy for obesity was first described in 1982,[3] and the Garren-Edwards gastric bubble (GEGB), an endoscopically-placed air-filled balloon, was approved for use by the FDA in 1985. However, multiple adverse events were reported with this device, including gastric mucosal injury, small bowel obstruction following spontaneous balloon deflation and migration, and poor efficacy compared with lifestyle modification alone in several trials.[4–11] The GEGB was withdrawn from the US market in 1992. Several design flaws likely contributed to its ultimate failure. It was made from polyurethane, which deflated too easily, and had a cylindrical shape with edges, which led to mucosal injury.[12] Additionally, it filled only to a volume of 220 mL, whereas a volume of 400 mL has been shown to be the minimum necessary to reduce food intake.[13] Subsequent efforts to design IGBs have drawn from the experience with the GEGB to create safer and more effective devices.[14,15] This article focuses on the IGBs that are available in the United States or for which pivotal trials are either ongoing or planned in the United States. Devices are summarized in **Table 1**.

Fluid-filled single balloon: Orbera

The most-studied and widely used IGB is the Orbera IGB, which was introduced in 1991 and originally known as the BioEnterics Intragastric Balloon (BIB, Allergan, Irvine,

Table 1
Intragastric balloons approved for use or being studied in the United States for Food and Drug Administration approval

Device Name	Structure/Materials	Fill Type and Volume	Method for Placing and Removing	Dwell Time
Orbera (Apollo Endosurgery)	Single silicone balloon	400–700 mL saline	Endoscopic	6 mo
ReShape Duo (ReShape Medical)	Two tethered silicone balloons	750 or 900 mL saline	Endoscopic	6 mo
Spatz (Spatz Medical)	Single silicone balloon, attached catheter	400–1000 mL saline, adjustable	Endoscopic	12 mo
Obalon (Obalon Therapeutics)	Lightweight balloon enclosed in capsule	250 mL gas, can swallow up to 3 balloons	Swallowed, removed endoscopically	6 mo
Elipse (Allurion Technologies)	Lightweight balloon enclosed in capsule	550 mL saline	Swallowed, degrades, passes in stool	4 mo

California) (**Fig. 1**). The Orbera IGB is a single spherical balloon made of silicone that is placed endoscopically and filled with saline. The deflated elastic balloon with attached catheter is passed into the stomach alongside a standard upper endoscope, and position in the body is confirmed by direct visualization. The device is then inflated with 400 to 700 mL of saline, often with 2 to 10 mL of methylene blue solution added. The methylene blue serves to alert the patient if the balloon has deflated; it is absorbed systemically and excreted in the urine, turning the urine green–blue in color.[16,17] The device remains in place for 6 months and is removed endoscopically. The Orbera balloon was approved by the FDA for treatment of obesity in 2015.

Recent meta-analyses have been conducted to evaluate efficacy and safety of the device. The ASGE Bariatric Endoscopy Task Force systematically reviewed 82 studies in 2015. Seventeen of these studies reported percent excess weight loss (%EWL) at 12 months after device implantation, or 6 months after removal, with a total of 1638 patients studied. These patients averaged a 25.4% EWL, with a 95% confidence interval (CI) of 21.5% to 29.4%. Only 3 studies had adequate control groups, with Orbera patients (n = 131) losing an average of 26.9% more weight than control patients (n = 95), with 95% CI of 15.6% to 38.2%.[18] A large randomized controlled trial has been conducted in the United States, but the results have not yet been published.

The Orbera balloon has also been well studied with respect to safety. In the ASGE task force meta-analysis, 68 studies reported rates of adverse events. Pain and nausea were most common, occurring in 33.7% of patients, with a 7% rate of early removal. More serious complications were rare, with ulceration in 2% of patients, migration in 1.4% of patients, small bowel obstruction of 0.3% of patients, and gastric perforation in 0.1% of patients. Four total deaths were reported, related to perforation or aspiration.[18] Most studies did not report timing of adverse events,[15] but in 1 larger retrospective series, 51 balloon leaks or deflations were observed, with 49 of these occurring after the recommended 6-month period.[19]

Fluid-filled dual balloon: ReShape duo

The ReShape Integrated Dual Balloon System is an endoscopically placed device consisting of 2 equal-sized silicone balloons connected by a flexible shaft (**Fig. 2**). After placement of the deflated dual-balloon device, each balloon is filled separately with either 375 or 450 mL of saline with methylene blue, for a total volume of 750 or

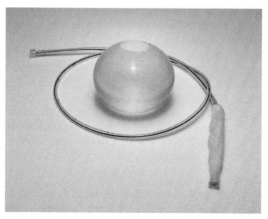

Fig. 1. Orbera balloon. (*Courtesy of* Apollo Endosurgery, Austin TX; with permission.)

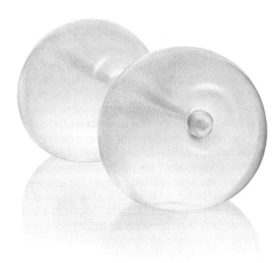

Fig. 2. ReShape integrated dual balloon system. (*Courtesy of* ReShape Medical, San Clemente, CA; with permission.)

900 mL depending on the height of the patient. This design is intended to prevent migration of the device, since unintentional deflation of 1 balloon would leave the other still intact and holding the device in place. The device is removed endoscopically at 6 months. ReShape was approved by the FDA for treatment of obesity in 2015.

The ReShape IGB was evaluated in the REDUCE (A Prospective, Randomized Multicenter Study to Evaluate the Safety and Efficacy of the ReShape Duo Intragastric Balloon System in Obese Subjects) randomized sham-controlled pivotal trial. The completed study included 326 participants with BMI 30 to 40 kg/m^2 at 8 US study centers, and all subjects received monthly lifestyle therapy coaching. At 24 weeks, Duo subjects had an average %EWL of 25.1% compared with 11.3% in Diet patients (P = .004) on intention-to-treat analysis.[20] An average of 66% of weight lost at time of balloon removal was maintained 24 weeks later.

Like other IGBs, abdominal pain, nausea, and vomiting were common, particularly in the first week after implantation. Early retrieval for intolerance occurred in 9% of patients within the first 2 months, which prompted a reduction in fill volume to 375 mL per balloon for patients shorter than 5 feet 4 inches tall, with subsequent reduction in early retrievals. In addition, gastric ulceration was seen in 39% of treatment patients, resulting in a minor design change to smooth the device tip, which reduced the ulcer rate to only 10%; most ulcers were noted incidentally on 6 month balloon removal. Deflation occurred in 6% of patients, with no migrations or obstructions observed.[20]

A subsequent clinical case series in Spain demonstrated 15.4% total body weight loss (TBWL) at 6 months in 60 patients. Only 1 early removal for intolerance occurred, and 1 leak occurred. Fourteen patients had ulcerations on balloon removal, and 1 patient had a gastric perforation. Of note, the old balloon design with higher rate of ulceration was used in all of these patients.[21]

Fluid-filled adjustable balloon: Spatz

The Spatz Adjustable Balloon System (Spatz Medical, Great Neck, New York) is an endoscopically placed, saline-filled single intragastric balloon (**Fig. 3**). Unlike other available IGBs, which are inflated to desired volume on implantation, the Spatz has

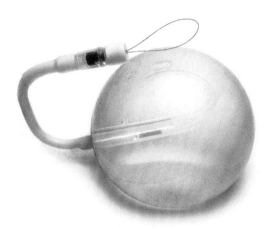

Fig. 3. Spatz balloon. (*Courtesy of* Spatz Medical, Great Neck, NY; with permission.)

an attached inflation tube that remains in the stomach with the balloon and can be extracted out through the mouth to adjust the balloon volume during therapy to improve tolerance or efficacy. The Spatz balloon is not approved by the FDA but is approved in Europe for 12 months of therapy.

At present, there are limited safety and efficacy data on the Spatz IGB. A study of 73 patients in the United Kingdom showed a 45.7% EWL. Four patients had the balloon removed due to intolerance; 10 patients had the volume adjusted downward with comparable weight loss outcomes, and 45 patients had the volume adjusted upward for decline in weight loss with mostly good efficacy. Complications included catheter migration and impaction resulting in need for surgical extraction in 3 cases,[22] which led to a change in the device design with a softer catheter. No difference in weight loss was seen in an 80-patient case–control study between 12 months of Spatz IGB and 12 months of Orbera treatment using 2 sequential balloons.[23] Safety concerns have been raised, with higher overall rates of complications compared with Orbera[23] and reports of delayed gastric or bowel perforation,[24–26] but the frequency of such complications is not yet known.

Gas-filled swallowed balloon: Obalon
The Obalon Gastric Balloon (OGB, Obalon Therapeutics, Carlsbad, California) differs from the previously discussed IGBs in that it is enclosed in a gelatin capsule, which is swallowed by the patient under fluoroscopic visualization (**Fig. 4**). The capsule has an attached catheter that extends through the esophagus and out of the mouth, and is used to inflate the balloon with 250 mL of a nitrogen-mix gas. A pilot study involving 17 patients was undertaken in Europe, with up to 3 balloons given per patient, swallowed individually at 4-week intervals, and removed endoscopically at 12 weeks. Average excess weight loss at 12 weeks was 36%, with no serious adverse events reported. Most patients experienced transient abdominal pain and nausea after balloon administration.[27] A large randomized sham-controlled trial in the United States with balloons in place for 6 months has recently been completed, but results have not yet been published.

Fluid-filled swallowed balloon: Elipse
The Elipse IGB (Allurion Technologies, Wellesley, Massachusetts) is enclosed within a capsule with an attached catheter and swallowed under radiographic guidance (**Fig. 5**). After placement is confirmed, the balloon is filled with 550 mL of fluid and

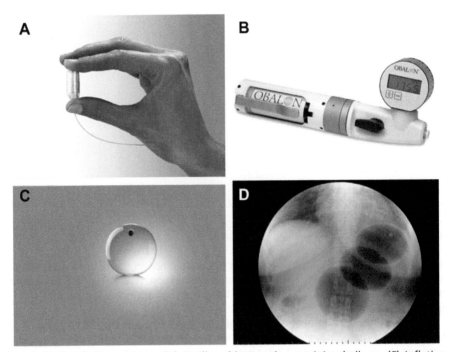

Fig. 4. Obalon Balloon System. (*A*) Swallowable capsule-containing balloon. (*B*) Inflation device. (*C*) Gas-filled balloon. (*D*) Radiograph of 3 deployed balloons in vivo. (*Courtesy of* Obalon Therapeutics, Carlsbad, CA; with permission.)

remains in the stomach for 4 months. The balloon is made with a material that degrades over the 4-month period on the internal side of the release valve. Once the material degrades, the release valve opens, causing a catastrophic deflation of the balloon, which then passes on its own. An 8-patient pilot study using a prototype demonstrated no adverse events other than nausea, vomiting, and cramping, and patients lost an average of 12.4% of excess weight over 6 weeks.[28] Results of a small multicenter study were reported at a recent conference, but have not yet been published.

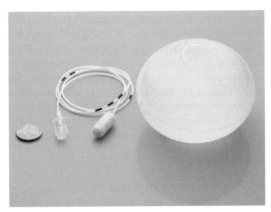

Fig. 5. Ellipse balloon. (*Courtesy of* Allurion Technologies, Wellesley, MA; with permission.)

TransPyloric Shuttle

The TransPyloric Shuttle (BAROnova, Goleta, California) consists of a spherical bulb attached by a flexible cord to a smaller cylindrical bulb (**Fig. 6**). The device is placed endoscopically and assembled in the stomach. The large bulb rests in the antrum, with the smaller bulb crossing into the duodenum. This creates intermittent obstruction at the pylorus leading to delayed gastric emptying and longer periods of satiety. One study of 20 participants showed promising results, with mean EWL of 25% at 3 months and 41% at 6 months and gastric ulcers in 50% of patients with early device removal in 2 patients due to symptomatic gastric ulcers.[29] The ENDObesity II multicenter study is currently underway, with no results yet published.

Tissue Apposition

Endoscopic sleeve gastroplasty

In endoscopic sleeve gastroplasty (ESG), gastric volume is reduced by using endo-scopically placed sutures to create a gastric sleeve similar to a sleeve gastrectomy. This is accomplished using the Overstitch endoscopic suturing device (Apollo Endo-surgery), an FDA-approved commercial device for the purposes of tissue apposition compatible with a double-channel therapeutic gastroscope (**Fig. 7**). Full-thickness stitches can be placed in interrupted or running patterns and sutures reloaded without removal of the endoscope.[16] The sleeve is created by apposing the gastric wall along the greater curvature.

The technique was first described in a pilot study involving 4 patients in 2013, which demonstrated the technical feasibility of such an approach.[30] In 2015, midterm results of an open-label trial were reported, with 25 patients (BMI 35.5) enrolled. Procedure time decreased from 217 minutes to 98 minutes when comparing the first 5 cases with the last 5 cases. All ESGs remained intact by endoscopic evaluation at 3 months, and patients had lost an average of 41% of excess body weight at 20 months.[31] Another study with 50 patients also demonstrated effective weight loss without serious adverse events, with the additional finding that increased contacts with nutritional and psycho-logical providers predicted successful weight loss at 1 year after the procedure.[32,33]

Primary Obesity Surgery Endoluminal

The Primary Obesity Surgery Endoluminal (POSE) procedure uses an overtube-style incisionless operating platform (USGI Medical, San Clemente, California) with

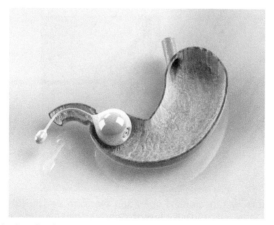

Fig. 6. Transpyloric shuttle. (*Courtesy of* BAROnova, Goleta, CA; with permission.)

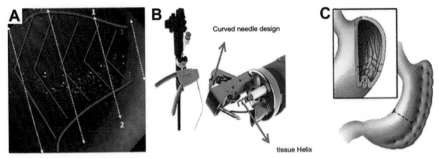

Fig. 7. Endoscopic sleeve gastroplasty. (*A*) Suturing pattern used. (*B*) Endoscopic suturing device (Apollo Overstitch). (*C*) Depiction of procedure. (*From* Abu Dayyeh BK, Acosta A, Camilleri M, et al. Endoscopic sleeve gastroplasty alters gastric physiology and induces loss of body weight in obese individuals. Clin Gastroenterol Hepatol 2015. [Epub ahead of print]; with permission.)

4working channels and accommodates a slim endoscope along with specialized instruments that are FDA-approved for tissue apposition (**Fig. 8**). Transmural tissue anchor plications are placed to reduce accommodation of the gastric fundus, with additional plications in the distal gastric body to delay emptying.

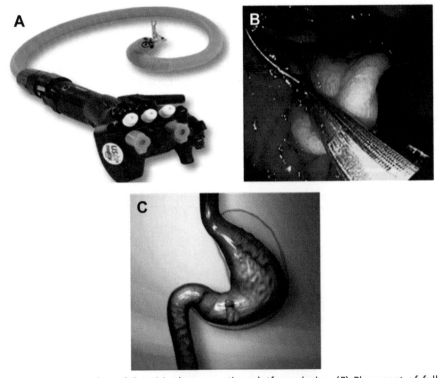

Fig. 8. POSE procedure. (*A*) Incisionless operating platform device. (*B*) Placement of full-thickness anchors in stomach. (*C*) Depiction of stomach following procedure. (*Courtesy of* USGI Medical, San Clemente, CA; with permission.)

Feasibility and safety were demonstrated in a single-center, open-label prospective trial in Spain with 45 patients evaluated, with 49% EWL average at 6 months.[34] Eighteen patients were evaluated to assess for physiologic changes related to weight loss, and were found to have significantly decreased intake capacity, initially delayed gastric emptying that returned to baseline by 6 months, improved insulin sensitivity, and enhanced postprandial decrease in ghrelin.[35] This approach was evaluated in the recently completed large multicenter randomized sham-controlled trial in the United States, the ESSENTIAL (A Randomized, Subject and Evaluator-Blinded, Parallel-Group, Multicenter Clinical Trial Using an Endoscopic Suturing Device [G-Cath EZ Suture Anchor Delivery Catheter] for Primary Weight Loss) trial; and a small multicenter randomized controlled trial in Europe, the MILEPOST (Multicenter Study of an Incisionless Operating Platform for Primary Obesity vs Diet and Exercise) study. Results have been presented in abstract form, but have not been published.

Nutrient-Diverting Therapy

Aspiration therapy

Aspiration therapy is a new endoscopic approach that involves placement of a large percutaneous silicone gastrostomy tube (A-Tube) that is subsequently connected with a skin port to an Aspire Assist device (Aspire Bariatrics, King of Prussia, Pennsylvania) **(Fig. 9)**. Following meal consumption, the patient uses this system to siphon off a portion of the ingested meal, typically one-third of the volume.

In a small pilot study published in 2013, patients in the aspiration group lost an average of 49% of excess weight, compared with 14.9% in the lifestyle therapy group. Weight loss was maintained at 2-year follow-up. No serious adverse effects were observed, and no binge eating episodes occurred.[36] Similar results were obtained in a single-arm prospective trial in Sweden.[37] A pivotal multicenter randomized controlled trial has been completed in the United States and presented at a recent meeting, but results have not yet been published.[38]

Duodenal–jejunal bypass liner

Because of the important role of the proximal small intestine in absorption of nutrients, endoscopic treatments have been developed to bypass this region using liners. The Endobarrier (GI Dynamics, Lexington, Massachusetts) is a 65 cm Teflon sleeve that is anchored in the duodenal bulb by a barbed nitinol crown **(Fig. 10)**. The device is placed under endoscopic and fluoroscopic guidance, and removed endoscopically at 12 months.

Efficacy has been assessed over several studies, with EWL ranging from 30% to 47% at 52 weeks.[17] The device also appears to have efficacy in improving glycemic

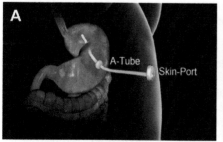
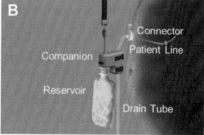

Fig. 9. Aspiration therapy. (*A*) A-tube. (*B*) Aspire Assist device. (*Courtesy of* Aspire Bariatrics, King of Prussia, PA; with permission.)

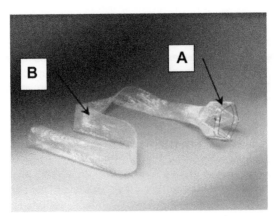

Fig. 10. Duodenal–jejunal bypass liner. (A) Anchor. (B) Liner. (*From* Escalona A, Yanez R, Pimentel F, et al. Initial human experience with restrictive duodenal–jejunal bypass liner for treatment of morbid obesity. Surg Obes Relat Dis 2010;6(2):127; with permission.)

control, insulin resistance, and lipid profile.[39] A recent meta-analysis found that patients had an average of 12.6% EWL with EndoBarrier compared to dietary modification, with an average of 0.9% change in glycated hemoglobin that failed to meet statistical significance.[40]

Common adverse effects of Endobarrier implantation in 271 patients from a literature review include abdominal pain, nausea, and vomiting;18% of patients required early removal. Device migration, GI bleeding, obstruction, and abdominal pain have been reasons cited for early removal.[40] Rare serious adverse events including esophageal perforation, cholangitis, and liver abscess have been reported.[17] A multicenter randomized sham-controlled pivotal trial in the United States, the ENDO (Safety and Efficacy of EndoBarrier in Subjects With Type 2 Diabetes Who Are Obese) trial, was stopped due to the incidence of liver abscess.

Gastroduodenojejunal bypass liner

A longer 120 cm fluoropolymer sleeve has been developed (ValenTx, Hopkins, Minnesota) that is secured at the gastroesophageal junction by a combined endoscopic and laparoscopic approach. The device bypasses the stomach, duodenum, and proximal jejunum. It is also left in place for 12 months and retrieved endoscopically. A 1-year prospective series with 12 patients enrolled showed an average EWL of 35.9%, with improvement in diabetes, hypertension, and hyperlipidemia, although 2 patients had the device removed due to dysphagia and odynophagia, and 4 patients were found to have partially detached devices at 12 months, with inferior weight loss results. No bowel erosions, ulcerations, or cases of pancreatitis were observed in this cohort.[41] A modification of this device that does not require laparoscopic assistance is being developed.[17]

Incisionless anastomosis system

Techniques have been developed to endoscopically deliver magnets to adjacent GI lumens, creating entero-enteral bypass anastomoses by magnetic compression. This concept has been applied in a small human study for treatment of malignant gastric outlet obstruction.[42] The incisionless anastomosis system (IAS, GI Windows, Boston, Massachusetts), previously known as self-assembling magnets for endoscopy (SAMSEN), consists of smart magnets that are delivered endoscopically in a linear configuration and form an octagonal shape intraluminally[43] (**Fig. 11**). When these are placed in opposing lumens, magnetic compression creates a large-bore

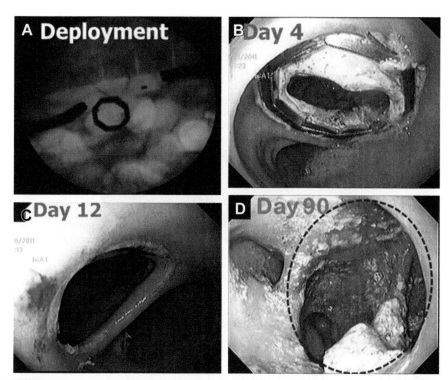

Fig. 11. Incisionless anastomosis system. (*A*) Fluoroscopic image of aligned magnets. (*B*) Colonoscopic image of coupled magnets causing ischemic necrosis. (*C*) Magnets spontaneously expelled. (*D*) Fully re-epithelialized, patent anastomosis. (*From* Ryou M, Agoston AT, Thompson CC. Endoscopic intestinal bypass creation by using self-assembling magnets in a porcine model. Gastrointest Endosc 2016;83(4):823; with permission.)

anastomosis that has been shown to be durable in a porcine model.[44] The process takes several days, during which time the magnets fuse, slough off from the mucosa, and pass without intervention; no obstructions or retained magnets occurred in a porcine study.[43] For bariatric use, this device may induce ileal break with decreased food intake and improved diabetic control.[45] This system has recently been evaluated in people in a feasibility study in Europe, but the results have not been published yet.

Mucosal resurfacing
The Revita duodenal mucosal resurfacing procedure (Fractyl Laboratories, Cambridge, Massachusetts) involves the use of radiofrequency ablation following saline lift to induce mucosal remodeling (**Fig. 12**). This may result in changes in enteroendocrine cells improving diabetic control. A pilot study has been completed, and a multicenter clinical trial is currently underway in Europe.

SECONDARY THERAPY

RYGB results in up to 70% excess weight loss after 2 years.[17,46–48] Patients can experience less-than-ideal weight loss or weight regain following bypass.[47,49] Weight regain after RYGB is not well understood; however, gastrojejunostomy anastomosis diameter has been associated with weight regain.[50] EBT techniques offer alternatives to surgical revision for treatment of weight regain after bypass or less-than-ideal weight loss.

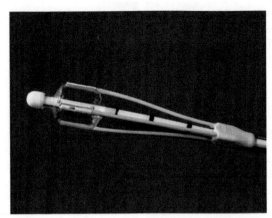

Fig. 12. Revita catheter for mucosal resurfacing. (*Courtesy of* Fractyl Laboratories, Cambridge, MA; with permission.)

Transoral Outlet Reduction

Transoral outlet reduction (TORe) is an endoscopic suturing technique that permits approximation of luminal tissue without incisions (**Fig. 13**). The RESTORe (Randomized Evaluation of Endoscopic Suturing Transorally for Anastomotic Outlet Reduction)

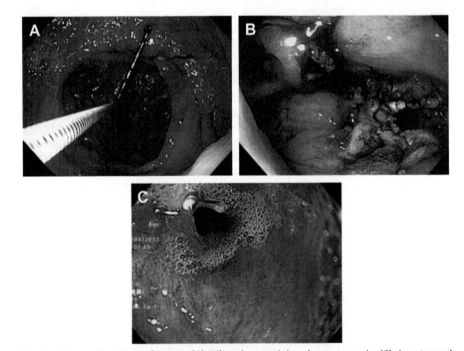

Fig. 13. Transoral outlet reduction. (*A*) Dilated gastrojejunal anastomosis. (*B*) Anastomosis following transoral outlet reduction using full-thickness suture device. (*C*) Anastomosis 6 months after procedure. (*From* Kumar N, Thompson CC. Comparison of a superficial suturing device with a full-thickness suturing device for transoral outlet reduction. Gastrointest Endosc 2014;79(6):986; with permission.)

trial compared TORe with sham treatment in RYGB patients with a gastrojejunal (GJ) anastomotic diameter greater than 2 cm with inadequate weight loss (failure to achieve 50% EWL) or weight regain (more than 5% EWL from nadir) using a partial-thickness suturing device (EndoCinch, C.R. Bard, Murray Hill, New Jersey). After 6 months, the TORe group had 3.5% total body weight loss compared with 0.4% in the control group. Ninety-six percent of patients had either weight loss or no further weight gain. No serious device-related adverse events were reported in the early post-procedure period.[51]

Subsequent data have emerged with a full-thickness suturing device, the Apollo Over-stitch (Apollo Endosurgery) (see **Fig. 7**). A prospective study by Kumar and colleagues[52] showed that endoscopic revision of dilated GJ anastomosis in 150 patients resulted in 9.5 plus or minus 2.1 kg or 19.2% plus or minus 4.6% EWL at 3 years after revision.

In addition to GJ stoma revision, TORe has also been associated with resolution of dumping and bile-associated reflux symptoms in patients with RYGB. Leitman and colleagues[53] performed TORe in 66 patients for severe dumping syndrome and re-ported resolution in 71% of patients with symptomatic improvement in all patients. The same study also reported resolution of severe reflux in 20% of patients and symp-tomatic improvement in 80% of patients.

Revision Obesity Surgery Endoscopic

The revision obesity surgery endoscopic (ROSE) procedure uses the Incisionless Operating Platform (IOP, USGI Medical) to place durable tissue anchors in the gastric lumen to create plications (see **Fig. 8**). In 2009, a multicenter prospective single-arm study of 116 patients using the ROSE procedure reported 69% of patients experi-enced increased satiety; 88% of patients stopped weight regain at 6 months, and 53% of patients achieved an EWL of at least 20%, with a mean 11.3 kg weight loss at 6 months. No significant complications occurred.[54–56]

Argon Plasma Coagulation

Argon plasma coagulation (APC) used with 65 to 75 W and 2-3 L/m flow can be used on the mucosa in the GJ anastomosis, leading to fibrosis of gastric mucosa and sub-sequent reduction of the GJ stoma. In a study of 215 patients by Sander and col-leagues, APC was used to decrease the diameter of the GJ stoma by almost 50% using an average of 1.36 sessions. Patients experienced on average 13.8 kg weight loss after the final APC session. However, 69 patients (32.1%) did not achieve the target stoma diameter. The main complication reported was symptomatic stenosis in 16.3% of patients, necessitating balloon dilation.[57]

SUMMARY

Multiple EBTs are currently being used in the United States for primary obesity treatment and treatment of weight regain after RYGB, and several studies have shown benefit with large randomized sham-controlled and nonsham-controlled designs. Multiple EBTs are under review by the FDA or are in the investigational phase for FDA approval. EBT should be used in conjunction with at least moderate-intensity lifestyle therapy as part of a comprehensive long-term weight management program for maximal benefit.

REFERENCES

1. Farina MG, Baratta R, Nigro A, et al. Intragastric balloon in association with lifestyle and/or pharmacotherapy in the long-term management of obesity. Obes Surg 2012;22(4):565–71.

2. Sullivan S, Kumar N, Edmundowicz SA, et al. ASGE position statement on endoscopic bariatric therapies in clinical practice. Gastrointest Endosc 2015;82(5): 767–72.
3. Nieben OG, Harboe H. Intragastric balloon as an artificial bezoar for treatment of obesity. Lancet 1982;1(8265):198–9.
4. Benjamin SB. Small bowel obstruction and the Garren-Edwards gastric bubble: an iatrogenic bezoar. Gastrointest Endosc 1988;34(6):463–7.
5. Benjamin SB, Maher KA, Cattau EL Jr, et al. Double-blind controlled trial of the Garren-Edwards gastric bubble: an adjunctive treatment for exogenous obesity. Gastroenterology 1988;95(3):581–8.
6. Hogan RB, Johnston JH, Long BW, et al. A double-blind, randomized, sham-controlled trial of the gastric bubble for obesity. Gastrointest Endosc 1989; 35(5):381–5.
7. Kirby DF, Wade JB, Mills PR, et al. A prospective assessment of the Garren-Edwards Gastric Bubble and bariatric surgery in the treatment of morbid obesity. Am surgeon 1990;56(10):575–80.
8. Lindor KD, Hughes RW Jr, Ilstrup DM, et al. Intragastric balloons in comparison with standard therapy for obesity—a randomized, double-blind trial. Mayo Clin Proc 1987;62(11):992–6.
9. Meshkinpour H, Hsu D, Farivar S. Effect of gastric bubble as a weight reduction device: a controlled, crossover study. Gastroenterology 1988;95(3):589–92.
10. Zeman RK, Benjamin SB, Cunningham MB, et al. Small bowel obstruction due to Garren gastric bubble: radiographic diagnosis. AJR Am J roentgenol 1988; 150(3):581–2.
11. Ziessman HA, Collen MJ, Fahey FH, et al. The effect of the Garren-Edwards Gastric Bubble on solid and liquid gastric emptying. Clin Nucl Med 1988;13(8): 586–9.
12. Sullivan S. Endoscopy in the management of obesity. Gastrointest Endosc Clin N Am 2013;23(1):165–75.
13. Geliebter A, Westreich S, Gage D. Gastric distention by balloon and test-meal intake in obese and lean subjects. Am J Clin Nutr 1988;48(3):592–4.
14. Schapiro M, Benjamin S, Blackburn G, et al. Obesity and the gastric balloon: a comprehensive workshop. Tarpon Springs, Florida, March 19-21, 1987. Gastrointest Endosc 1987;33(4):323–7.
15. Gaur S, Levy S, Mathus-Vliegen L, et al. Balancing risk and reward: a critical review of the intragastric balloon for weight loss. Gastrointest Endosc 2015;81(6): 1330–6.
16. Kumar N. Endoscopic therapy for weight loss: gastroplasty, duodenal sleeves, intragastric balloons, and aspiration. World J Gastrointest Endosc 2015;7(9): 847–59.
17. Abu Dayyeh BK, Edmundowicz SA, Jonnalagadda S, et al. Endoscopic bariatric therapies. Gastrointest Endosc 2015;81(5):1073–86.
18. Force ABET, Committee AT, Abu Dayyeh BK, et al. ASGE Bariatric Endoscopy Task Force systematic review and meta-analysis assessing the ASGE PIVI thresholds for adopting endoscopic bariatric therapies. Gastrointest Endosc 2015; 82(3):425–438 e425.
19. Roman S, Napoleon B, Mion F, et al. Intragastric balloon for "non-morbid" obesity: a retrospective evaluation of tolerance and efficacy. Obes Surg 2004;14(4): 539–44.

20. Ponce J, Woodman G, Swain J, et al. The REDUCE pivotal trial: a prospective, randomized controlled pivotal trial of a dual intragastric balloon for the treatment of obesity. Surg Obes Relat Dis 2015;11(4):874–81.
21. Lopez-Nava G, Bautista-Castano I, Jimenez-Banos A, et al. Dual intragastric balloon: single ambulatory center Spanish experience with 60 patients in endoscopic weight loss management. Obes Surg 2015;25(12):2263–7.
22. Brooks J, Srivastava ED, Mathus-Vliegen EM. One-year adjustable intragastric balloons: results in 73 consecutive patients in the U.K. Obes Surg 2014;24(5): 813–9.
23. Genco A, Dellepiane D, Baglio G, et al. Adjustable intragastric balloon vs non-adjustable intragastric balloon: case-control study on complications, tolerance, and efficacy. Obes Surg 2013;23(7):953–8.
24. Al-Zubaidi AM, Alghamdi HU, Alzobydi AH, et al. Bowel perforation due to break and distal passage of the safety ring of an adjustable intra-gastric balloon: a potentially life threatening situation. World J Gastrointest Endosc 2015;7(4): 429–32.
25. Daniel F, Abou Fadel C, Houmani Z, et al. Spatz 3 adjustable intragastric balloon: long-term safety concerns. Obes Surg 2016;26(1):159–60.
26. Dayan D, Sagie B, Fishman S. Late intragastric balloon induced gastric perforation. Obes Surg 2016;26(5):1138–40.
27. Mion F, Ibrahim M, Marjoux S, et al. Swallowable Obalon(R) gastric balloons as an aid for weight loss: a pilot feasibility study. Obes Surg 2013;23(5):730–3.
28. Machytka E, Chuttani R, Bojkova M, et al. Elipse, a procedureless gastric balloon for weight loss: a proof-of-concept pilot study. Obes Surg 2016;26(3):512–6.
29. Marinos G, Eliades C, Raman Muthusamy V, et al. Weight loss and improved quality of life with a nonsurgical endoscopic treatment for obesity: clinical results from a 3- and 6-month study. Surg Obes Relat Dis 2014;10(5):929–34.
30. Abu Dayyeh BK, Rajan E, Gostout CJ. Endoscopic sleeve gastroplasty: a potential endoscopic alternative to surgical sleeve gastrectomy for treatment of obesity. Gastrointest Endosc 2013;78(3):530–5.
31. Abu Dayyeh BK, Acosta A, Camilleri M, et al. Endoscopic sleeve gastroplasty alters gastric physiology and induces loss of body weight in obese individuals. Clin Gastroenterol Hepatol 2015. [Epub ahead of print].
32. Lopez-Nava G, Galvao M, Bautista-Castano I, et al. Endoscopic sleeve gastroplasty with 1-year follow-up: factors predictive of success. Endosc Int open 2016;4(2):E222–7.
33. Lopez-Nava G, Galvao MP, Bautista-Castano I, et al. Endoscopic sleeve gastroplasty: how I do it? Obes Surg 2015;25(8):1534–8.
34. Espinos JC, Turro R, Mata A, et al. Early experience with the incisionless operating platform (IOP) for the treatment of obesity : the primary obesity surgery endolumenal (POSE) procedure. Obes Surg 2013;23(9):1375–83.
35. Espinos JC, Turro R, Moragas G, et al. Gastrointestinal physiological changes and their relationship to weight loss following the POSE procedure. Obes Surg 2016;26(5):1081–9.
36. Sullivan S, Stein R, Jonnalagadda S, et al. Aspiration therapy leads to weight loss in obese subjects: a pilot study. Gastroenterology 2013;145(6):1245–52.e1-5.
37. Forssell H, Noren E. A novel endoscopic weight loss therapy using gastric aspiration: results after 6 months. Endoscopy 2015;47(1):68–71.
38. Thompson CC, Dayyeh BKA, Kushner R, et al. 381 The AspireAssist Is an Effective Tool in the Treatment of Class II and Class III Obesity: Results of a One-Year Clinical Trial. Gastroenterology 2016;150:S86.

39. Jain D, Singhal S. Endoscopic bypass using endobarrier devices: efficacy in treating obesity and metabolic syndrome. J Clin Gastroenterol 2015;49(10): 799–803.

40. Rohde U, Hedback N, Gluud LL, et al. Effect of the endobarrier gastrointestinal liner on obesity and type 2 diabetes: a systematic review and meta-analysis. Diabetes Obes Metab 2016;18(3):300–5.

41. Sandler BJ, Rumbaut R, Swain CP, et al. One-year human experience with a novel endoluminal, endoscopic gastric bypass sleeve for morbid obesity. Surg Endosc 2015;29(11):3298–303.

42. Chopita N, Vaillaverde A, Cope C, et al. Endoscopic gastroenteric anastomosis using magnets. Endoscopy 2005;37(4):313–7.

43. Ryou M, Aihara H, Thompson CC. Minimally invasive entero-enteral dual-path bypass using self-assembling magnets. Surg Endosc 2016;30(10):4533–8.

44. Ryou M, Agoston AT, Thompson CC. Endoscopic intestinal bypass creation by using self-assembling magnets in a porcine model. Gastrointest Endosc 2016; 83(4):821–5.

45. Ryou M, Cantillon-Murphy P, Azagury D, et al. Smart Self-Assembling MagnetS for ENdoscopy (SAMSEN) for transoral endoscopic creation of immediate gastro-jejunostomy (with video). Gastrointest Endosc 2011;73(2):353–9.

46. Bour ES. Evidence supporting the need for bariatric surgery to address the obesity epidemic in the United States. Curr Sports Med Rep 2015;14(2):100–3.

47. Magro DO, Geloneze B, Delfini R, et al. Long-term weight regain after gastric bypass: a 5-year prospective study. Obes Surg 2008;18(6):648–51.

48. Buchwald H. The evolution of metabolic/bariatric surgery. Obes Surg 2014;24(8): 1126–35.

49. Karmali S, Brar B, Shi X, et al. Weight recidivism post-bariatric surgery: a systematic review. Obes Surg 2013;23(11):1922–33.

50. Abu Dayyeh BK, Lautz DB, Thompson CC. Gastrojejunal stoma diameter predicts weight regain after Roux-en-Y gastric bypass. Clin Gastroenterol Hepatol 2011; 9(3):228–33.

51. Thompson CC, Chand B, Chen YK, et al. Endoscopic suturing for transoral outlet reduction increases weight loss after Roux-en-Y gastric bypass surgery. Gastroenterology 2013;145(1):129–137 e123.

52. Kumar N, Thompson CC. Transoral outlet reduction for weight regain after gastric bypass: long-term follow-up. Gastrointest Endosc 2016;83(4):776–9.

53. Leitman IM, Virk CS, Avgerinos DV, et al. Early results of trans-oral endoscopic plication and revision of the gastric pouch and stoma following Roux-en-Y gastric bypass surgery. JSLS 2010;14(2):217–20.

54. Mullady DK, Lautz DB, Thompson CC. Treatment of weight regain after gastric bypass surgery when using a new endoscopic platform: initial experience and early outcomes (with video). Gastrointest Endosc 2009;70(3):440–4.

55. Horgan S, Jacobsen G, Weiss GD, et al. Incisionless revision of post-Roux-en-Y bypass stomal and pouch dilation: multicenter registry results. Surg Obes Relat Dis 2010;6(3):290–5.

56. Ryou M, Ryan MB, Thompson CC. Current status of endoluminal bariatric procedures for primary and revision indications. Gastrointest Endosc Clin N Am 2011; 21(2):315–33.

57. Sander BN, Neto MG, Baretta G, et al. Endoscopic revision with argon plasma coagulation for failed Roux-And-Y gastric bypass (Rygb). First large series. Surg Obes Relat Dis 2015;11(6):S29.

The Surgical Management of Obesity

Christopher J. Neylan, BA[a], Umashankkar Kannan, MD[b], Daniel T. Dempsey, MD[a], Noel N. Williams, MD[a], Kristoffel R. Dumon, MD[a],*

KEYWORDS

- Gastric bypass • Sleeve gastrectomy • Weight loss • Diabetes • Bariatric surgery
- Lap band

KEY POINTS

- Bariatric surgery is currently the best known treatment of obesity.
- The sleeve gastrectomy and Roux-en-Y gastric bypass are the two most popular bariatric operations.
- Bariatric surgery has the potential to improve multiple obesity-related comorbidities.

INTRODUCTION

Obesity (body mass index [BMI] $\geq$30 kg/m^2) remains a significant problem in the United States, as more than one-third of the American population is obese.[1] Obesity's burden on the nation's health care system can be quantified in terms of patient health as well health economics. With respect to the former, obesity is associated with a range of health issues, including diabetes, cancer, and heart disease.[2] Overweight-obesity is responsible for as many as 10% of deaths in America.[3]

At present, bariatric surgery is the best known treatment of obesity, and multiple meta-analyses have shown bariatric surgery to be more effective than diet and exercise or pharmacologic treatment.[4–6]

Bariatric surgery is marked by large and rapid growth over the last 2 decades. In 1998, 12,775 bariatric operations were performed in the United States. By 2004, that number increased to 135,985. The modern era of bariatric surgery began in 2005, which is defined by a drastic increase in the use of laparoscopy. Although in 2004 less than one-third of bariatric operations were performed laparoscopically, more than 97% of bariatric operations are now laparoscopic procedures.[7]

Disclosure: The authors have no disclosures.
[a] Department of Surgery, Hospital of the University of Pennsylvania, 3400 Spruce Street, Philadelphia, PA 19104, USA; [b] Department of Surgery, Bronx-Lebanon Hospital Center, 1650 Grand Concourse, Bronx, NY 10457, USA
* Corresponding author.
E-mail address: dumonk@uphs.upenn.edu

Gastroenterol Clin N Am 45 (2016) 689–703
http://dx.doi.org/10.1016/j.gtc.2016.07.006
0889-8553/16/© 2016 Elsevier Inc. All rights reserved.

gastro.theclinics.com

Three main procedures dominate bariatric surgery: the gastric bypass, sleeve gastrectomy, and gastric band. At their respective peaks, the gastric bypass (in 2003) accounted for 99% of all bariatric surgeries, the gastric band (in 2008) accounted for 29% of all bariatric operations, and the sleeve gastrectomy (in 2012) accounted for 42% of all bariatric operations.[7] **Fig. 1** shows trends in the distribution of bariatric procedures over time, from 2004 to 2012.

Patients who undergo bariatric operations are predominantly white and middle aged, and more than 80% are female. These patients have higher rates of obesity-related comorbidities, such as diabetes and hypertension, than the national average. The goal of bariatric surgery is to help patients lose weight and resolve comorbidities associated with obesity. This article reviews the state of bariatric surgery, with a particular emphasis on the relationship between bariatric surgery and gastrointestinal-related comorbidities.

CURRENT OPTIONS: BARIATRIC SURGERY

The 4 main bariatric procedures, along with their mechanisms of action, are shown in **Fig. 2**.

Gastric Bypass

The Roux-en-Y gastric bypass has been called the gold standard of bariatric surgery. Its effects are restrictive (reduction of stomach capacity), malabsorptive (decreased absorption by the digestive tract), and hormonal (changes in gut hormone levels).

Sleeve Gastrectomy

The sleeve gastrectomy is a common procedure in which the size of the stomach is reduced by approximately 75%, by resecting the greater curvature of the stomach. The sleeve gastrectomy has restrictive and hormonal effects.[8]

Adjustable Gastric Banding

The adjustable gastric band consists of a silicone band attached to an inflatable balloon, which is connected to an access port via a tube.[8,9] There are currently 2 FDA-approved gastric banding devices: the Lap-Band Gastric Banding System and the Realize Gastric Band.[10] This procedure is purely restrictive.

Biliopancreatic Diversion

Biliopancreatic diversion may be performed as a stand-alone operation, or it may be combined with a duodenal switch in a procedure called the biliopancreatic diversion with duodenal switch. Both procedures are described in detail elsewhere.[8,11,12] This procedure is restrictive, malabsorptive, and hormonal. It accounts for only about 2% of bariatric operations.[13]

ELIGIBILITY FOR BARIATRIC SURGERY

Bariatric surgery is currently recommended for patients with a BMI greater than or equal to 40 kg/m^2, or a BMI greater than or equal to 35 kg/m^2 with at least 1 serious obesity-related comorbidity, such as heart disease, type II diabetes mellitus (T2DM), or severe sleep apnea. Recently, the American Society of Metabolic and Bariatric Surgery (ASMBS) and the International Federation for the Surgery of Obesity and Metabolic Disorders (IFSO) have emphasized the importance of considering bariatric surgery for patients with BMI greater than or equal to 30 kg/m^2, provided that they also have serious obesity-related comorbidities. Recent evidence has emerged that

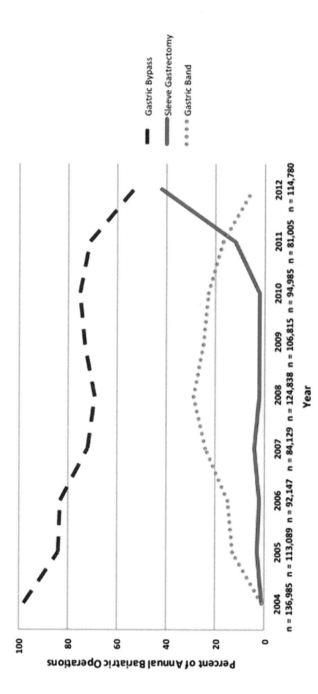

Fig. 1. Trends in the distribution of bariatric operations. The numbers listed below the years on the X axis indicate the total estimated number of bariatric operations performed that year in the United States. The numbers are taken from a national estimate that did not include biliopancreatic diversion.[7] Biliopancreatic diversion accounts for an additional 2% of bariatric procedures.[13] (*Data from* Nguyen NT, Vu S, Kim E, et al. Trends in utilization of bariatric surgery, 2009-2012. Surg Endosc 2016;30(7):2723–7; and Buchwald H, Oien DM. Metabolic/bariatric surgery worldwide 2011. Obes Surg 2013;23(4):427–36.)

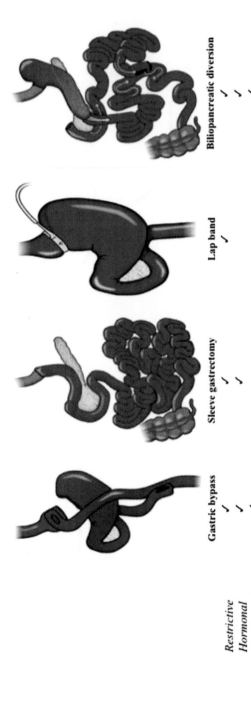

Restrictive
Hormonal
Malabsorptive

Fig. 2. The 4 bariatric procedures and their mechanisms of action.

supports the use of bariatric surgery in this patient population, and the FDA approved gastric banding for these patients. However, the Centers for Medicare and Medicaid Services do not approve coverage for patients with a BMI less than 35 kg/m^2.

WEIGHT LOSS

Current research supports the notion that bariatric surgery is the most effective treatment of obesity.[6] The mechanism of action for bariatric surgery has been described through use of the BRAVE (Bile flow alteration, Reduction of gastric size, Anatomic gut rearrangement and altered flow of nutrients, Vagal manipulation, and Enteric gut hormone modulation) effects.[14] The current theory behind weight loss following bariatric surgery attributes weight loss primarily to physiologic, rather than mechanical, changes. Reduction in levels of ghrelin and leptin, postprandial glucagon-like peptide-1 level increase, and peptide tyrosine tyrosine-response restoration are all credited with playing a major role in weight loss following gastric bypass, as are changes in the intestinal flora and bile acid levels.[15] The sleeve gastrectomy is thought to produce weight loss in similar ways, although the mechanism of action in the sleeve gastrectomy is not as well understood as it is in the gastric bypass.[16]

Gastric Banding

Gastric banding was initially a popular procedure. However, in the long term, many band-related complications have been reported, requiring band removal in almost 50% of patients.[17] Among those patients who have not had the band removed, reports of excess weight loss (EWL) range up to 50%, with follow-up between 5 and 15 years.[17] Compared with laparoscopic sleeve gastrectomy and Roux-en-Y gastric bypass, gastric banding has shown inferior weight loss results and a higher complication rate.[18]

Sleeve Gastrectomy

A systematic review involving 123 studies on the sleeve gastrectomy reported a 59% EWL 1 year after surgery, 64.5% 2 years after surgery, 66% 3 years after surgery, and 60.9% 4 years after surgery.[19] These results are similar to those reported in other systematic reviews.[20]

Roux-en-Y Gastric Bypass

Gastric bypass is traditionally considered the gold standard of bariatric surgery. A recent analysis of the long-term results of Roux-en-Y gastric bypass reported 57% EWL at 10 years of follow-up.[21] In a matched cohort study, gastric bypass showed superior EWL (67%) to both sleeve gastrectomy (56%) and gastric banding (44%).[22] This finding has been repeated elsewhere; for example, one study reported an EWL of 76% for the gastric bypass, 53% for sleeve gastrectomy, and 30% for the gastric band.[23]

Roux-en-Y Gastric Bypass Versus Sleeve Gastrectomy

One of the highest priority questions currently facing bariatric surgeons is whether or not the sleeve gastrectomy can replace the Roux-en-Y gastric bypass as the gold standard surgical procedure. The proven long-term success of the gastric bypass must be weighed against the technical complexity of the procedure and the associated risk for complications. One recent meta-analysis synthesized data from 62 studies comparing the Roux-en-Y gastric bypass with the sleeve gastrectomy (including several randomized controlled trials), resulting in data from 18,455 patients. After fitting a random-effects model, this study found that Roux-en-Y gastric bypass patients had a significantly higher percentage EWL (%EWL) than did sleeve gastrectomy patients, with a weighted mean difference of 7.24%.[24] Similarly, a separate meta-analysis found that gastric bypass patients had a higher 2-year postoperative %EWL following surgery as well as a lower 2-year postoperative BMI than did sleeve gastrectomy patients.[25]

SURVIVAL/MORTALITY

The in-hospital mortality of bariatric surgery is low. One recent study puts the number between 0.07% and 0.10%,[7] while another review cites the range of mortality as 0.1% to 2.0%.[26] A meta-analysis that included nearly 200,000 patients showed that patients who underwent bariatric surgery had greater than a 50% reduction in mortality relative to control patients who did not undergo surgery.[27] One study found that bariatric surgery patients gained an extra 6.5 years of life expectancy relative to a severely obese patient who did not undergo surgery.[28]

OUTCOMES: GASTROINTESTINAL RELATED
Gallbladder Disease

The relationship between bariatric surgery and gallbladder disease is complex, confounded significantly by the practice of prophylactic cholecystectomy (the routine removal of the gallbladder during bariatric surgery). Rapid weight loss is a risk factor for cholelithiasis, and approximately 35% to 38% of patients develop gallstones after bariatric surgery.[29] Some reports show that up to 40% of these patients become symptomatic,[29] which is often cited as a reason for prophylactic cholecystectomy. However, others claim that only 7% to 15% of patients who develop gallstones after bariatric surgery become symptomatic.[30] Thus the practice of prophylactic cholecystectomy during gastric bypass is controversial.[29] A recent Swedish study analyzing 13,443 patients suggested that the increased need for cholecystectomy following gastric bypass may be caused in part by increased detection caused by the bariatric operation itself, and concluded that prophylactic cholecystectomy may not be recommended.[31]

The American Society for Metabolic and Bariatric Surgery has recently recommended that normal and asymptomatic gallbladders not be removed at the time of surgery unless clinically indicated.

Nonalcoholic Fatty Liver Disease

Nonalcoholic fatty liver disease is one way that metabolic syndrome presents in the liver. It has an incidence of up to 70% in the obese,[32] and bariatric surgery significantly reduces histologic features (eg, steatosis and fibrosis) and enzyme levels associated with nonalcoholic fatty liver disease.[33]

Obesity and Gastroesophageal Reflux Disease

Gastroesophageal reflux disease (GERD) is a disease of the upper digestive tract that can significantly affect the quality of life of affected patients. In the general Western population, the incidence of GERD is approximately 10% to 20%.[34] This number increases significantly in the obese population (between 37% and 72% of obese patients have GERD), and some clinicians have suggested a causal link between obesity and GERD.[35] The impact that bariatric surgery has on GERD depends markedly on the procedure performed.

Roux-en-Y gastric bypass is superior to other procedures in improving GERD symptoms. Approximately 56.5% of patients with GERD reported improvement in their symptoms following gastric bypass.[36] It is thought that gastric bypass improves

GERD symptoms because of weight loss, the diversion of bile from the Roux limb, and reduced acid production (the small pouch created in the procedure lacks parietal cells).

Several studies find that there is an increase in the prevalence of GERD symptoms following sleeve gastrectomy, including a recent systematic review and meta-analysis.[35] It has been proposed that this occurs because of any or all of the follow mechanisms: a decline in lower esophageal sphincter pressure, the disruption of the angle of His, the decline in gastric compliance, and high intragastric pressure.[35] A significant number of studies have reported new-onset GERD following sleeve gastrectomy (ie, patients who did not have GERD before surgery develop it after surgery).[35] One proposed mechanism of action for this is that hiatal hernias develop following surgery and then the sleeve migrates above the level of the hiatus.[35]

The association of GERD with gastric banding is controversial. Multiple studies show an improvement in symptoms and decrease in medications related to GERD following banding.[37] A systematic review showed a decrease in reflux symptoms postoperatively, from 32.9% to 7.7%, as well as a decrease in medication usage, from 27.5% to 9.5%.[38] Other studies show an increase in GERD symptoms following gastric banding, and propose that the increase results from either esophageal dysmotility or esophageal outflow obstruction caused by increased pressure following band placement.[39]

If there is an onset or worsening of GERD after bariatric surgery, symptoms are treated initially with acid-reducing medications and promotility agents (as they would be in the general population). If medical therapy fails, then revisional surgery is considered. In the cases of gastric banding or sleeve gastrectomy, conversion to gastric bypass has successfully reduced GERD symptoms. In the case of gastric bypass, revisions include lengthening the Roux limb or downsizing the pouch that was created during the initial surgery.

Bariatric Surgery and Inflammatory Bowel Disease

Inflammatory bowel disease (IBD) is a term that refers collectively to 3 conditions: Crohn's disease, ulcerative colitis, and indeterminate colitis. Although IBD is not traditionally associated with obesity, current research suggests that obesity may play a role in inducing IBD and recent reports have shown that the prevalence of obesity among patients with IBD is increasing.[40]

Several technical considerations come into play when considering gut surgery on patients with IBD. Many surgeons do not to perform bariatric surgery on patients with IBD. Data are therefore scarce on the effects of bariatric surgery on IBD. However, one small study suggested that sleeve gastrectomy and gastric banding are safe in patients with IBD, and saw no exacerbation or only mild exacerbation of IBD symptoms following surgery.[41] Another study of 20 patients who underwent bariatric surgery reported that bariatric surgery is safe and effective in this patient population, and further that 90% of patients who were on pharmacotherapy to control their IBD-related symptoms experienced significant improvement in their symptoms and a major reduction in the maintenance medical therapy following surgery.[42]

OUTCOMES: NON–GASTROINTESTINAL RELATED
Metabolic Syndrome

The term metabolic syndrome refers to a series of biochemical and physiologic markers that collectively increase an individual's risk of heart disease, type 2 diabetes mellitus (T2DM), stroke, and a host of other health problems. An analysis of 4 randomized controlled trials found that patients who underwent bariatric surgery were more than twice as likely to achieve metabolic syndrome remission than were patients who did not undergo surgery.[6] Even when surgery patients were compared with patients who underwent intensive medical weight management, the surgery patients were still significantly more likely to achieve remission of metabolic syndrome.[43]

Cancer

The effect of bariatric surgery on cancer is not well established. Several studies have suggested that bariatric surgery decreases the risk of cancer, although this effect is seen mostly in women. However, recent studies have stated that, contrary to the risk of cancer being decreased following bariatric surgery, the risk of colorectal cancer may increase. These investigators have criticized the studies supporting a decreased risk of cancer following surgery as not meeting high standards of evidence.[44] One systematic review claims that 4 studies show a significantly decreased risk of colorectal cancer following surgery, relative to obese individuals who have not been operated on, but warns that these studies are not well designed.[44]

Diabetes and Bariatric Surgery

Patients with T2DM may benefit significantly from bariatric surgery, because many investigators have reported high remission rates (up to 78%) and a significant reduction in antidiabetic drugs following bariatric surgery, compared with medical weight management.[45] Further, one analysis of randomized controlled trials found that patients who underwent bariatric surgery were 22 times as likely to achieve diabetes remission as matched control patients who did not undergo surgery (when the data were analyzed using the conservative case scenario procedure rather than complete case analysis, surgery patients were 5 times as likely to achieve diabetes remission than nonsurgery patients).[6]

Schauer and colleagues[46] randomized 150 patients to 3 groups: intensive medical therapy, intensive medical therapy with sleeve gastrectomy, and intensive medical therapy with Roux-en-Y gastric bypass. At baseline, the average duration of T2DM in their patient population was 8.3 years, with 43% requiring insulin. The mean glycated hemoglobin A_1C (HbA_1C) was 9.3%. At 3 years, the target HbA_1C (6% or less) was achieved in 5% of patients in medical therapy group, 24% of patients in the sleeve gastrectomy group, and 38% of patients in the gastric bypass group.

Mingrone and colleagues[45,47] compared the effect of medical weight management on T2DM with the effect of bariatric surgery (either Roux-en-Y gastric bypass or biliopancreatic diversion with duodenal switch). Diabetes remission (defined as a fasting glucose level <100 mg/dL and glycated hemoglobin <6.5% for at least 1 year) at 2 years was not achieved in any medical weight management patients, but was achieved in 75% of the gastric bypass patients and 95% of the biliopancreatic diversion patients. At 5 years (88% follow-up), none of the patients in the medical group achieved diabetes remission, but 37% of the patients in the gastric bypass group and 63% of the patients in the biliopancreatic diversion group were in diabetes remission.

Compared with T2DM, bariatric surgery has a limited effect on type 1 diabetes mellitus. In a retrospective review involving 10 patients with type 1 diabetes and 20 matched patients with T2DM, with a follow-up of close to 5 years, the remission rate of patients with T2DM was 55%, compared with 0% for type 1 patients (although type 1 patients showed a 90% rate of improvement, and the remaining 45% of patients with T2DM showed improvement as well).[48]

Bariatric Surgery and Sleep Apnea

Obstructive sleep apnea is a condition in which the upper airway repeatedly partially or completely collapses during sleep. This condition affects more than 100 million adults in the United States, up to 58% of whom are affected by obesity. A recent study suggests that a 10% increase in body weight from baseline results in a 6-fold increase in risk for obstructive sleep apnea.[49] Among obese patients, weight loss is often recommended to treat sleep apnea.

A recent systematic review evaluated the effect of bariatric surgery on obstructive sleep apnea. On the whole, bariatric surgery had an excellent effect on sleep apnea, because more than 75% of patients had some improvement in their symptoms. Biliopancreatic diversion (with or without duodenal switch) was shown to have the best effect of all the bariatric operations, because 99% of these patients showed an improvement in their symptoms, and 82% had a resolution of sleep apnea. (The mean EWL in this group was 54%.) On average, 86% of sleeve gastrectomy patients showed resolution or improvement of their sleep apnea symptoms, and 79% of Roux-en-Y gastric bypass patients showed resolution or improvement. (The mean EWLs in these groups were 46% and 75%, respectively.) Laparoscopic adjustable gastric banding was the least effective among the bariatric procedures in improving sleep apnea, because 77% of patients showed resolution or improvement after surgery.[50]

Nutritional Deficiencies

The diets of obese individuals consist largely of high-fat and high-calorie foods with poor nutritional quality, predisposing obese patients to malnutrition.[51–53] Postoperative nutritional deficiencies are frequently seen in bariatric patients, and the extent of nutritional deficiency often correlates with the effectiveness of the procedure in promoting weight loss.[54]

The best-practice guidelines for nutritional supplements 3 to 6 months after bariatric surgery are presented in **Table 1**.[54]

Macronutrient deficiencies

Protein malnutrition is the major macronutrient deficiency seen after bariatric surgery. Biliopancreatic diversion (with or without duodenal switch) shows the highest rate of protein malnutrition: at 3% to 18%.[55] Hair loss is the first manifestation of protein malnutrition, followed by edema, emaciation, and biochemical findings of anemia

Table 1
Nutrition guidelines, less than or equal to 6 months postoperatively

Procedure	Minimal Required Daily Nutritional Supplements
Roux-en-Y gastric bypass, sleeve gastrectomy	2 adult multivitamin and mineral (containing iron, folate, and thiamine) supplements 1200–1500 mg of elemental calcium (in diet and as citrated supplements) + 3000 IU of vitamin D (titrated to 25-hydroxyvitamin D levels >30 ng/mL) Vitamin B_{12} (as needed to maintain normal levels) 45–60 mg of iron via multivitamins and additional supplements
Gastric banding	1 adult multivitamin and mineral (containing iron, folate, and thiamine) supplements 1200–1500 mg of elemental calcium (in diet and as citrated supplements) + 3000 IU of vitamin D (titrated to 25-hydroxyvitamin D levels >30 ng/mL)

and hypoalbuminemia.[56] A minimal protein intake of 60 g/d, and up to 1.5 to 2.1 g/kg of body weight per day, is recommended following surgery.[54]

Micronutrient deficiencies

Iron is the most common micronutrient deficiency following bariatric surgery, occurring in up to 50% of patients 4 years after gastric bypass.[57–59] However, this may be confounded by a high rate of preoperative iron deficiency.[60] A hypoacidic environment following gastric bypass, as well as the bypassing of absorption in the duodenum and proximal jejunum, contributes to iron deficiency.[61] Anemia is a major consequence of iron deficiency. Ferritin level, serum iron level, and total iron binding capacity should be measured 6 months after surgery to determine iron status and then measured annually.[54] Studies show that supplementing iron with vitamin C is significantly better than iron alone in treating iron deficiency.[62]

Other deficiencies

About 63% of patients develop vitamin D deficiency after surgery.[63,64] The consequences of vitamin D deficiency include hypocalcemia, secondary hyperparathyroidism, and parathyroid hormone–mediated cortical bone loss leading to metabolic bone disease.[64]

Vitamin A deficiency is seen in around 10% of patients 4 years after gastric bypass, and in 60% of patients following biliopancreatic diversion. Routine screening for vitamin A is recommended after surgery, and supplementation is indicated for deficiencies.[54] Vitamin A deficiency presents as night blindness or ocular xerosis, and is treated with 5000 to 10,000 IU/d until the vitamin A level normalizes. Vitamin E deficiency following bariatric surgery is uncommon.[63] There is insufficient evidence to routinely screen for vitamin E and K deficiencies.[54]

Thiamine deficiency can occur in up to 49% of patients following gastric bypass and 31% following sleeve gastrectomy, and is primarily caused by intractable vomiting following surgery.[65,66] Thiamine deficiency affects the nervous system, leading to beriberi, Korsakoff syndrome, and Wernicke encephalopathy. Routine screening is not recommended but should be considered in patients with rapid weight loss or intractable vomiting.[54] Other vitamin B deficiencies, including riboflavin, niacin, pantothenic acid, and biotin, are rare.[67]

Zinc deficiency is seen in 36% to 51% of post–bariatric surgery patients, and presents as a rash similar to acrodermatitis enteropathica.[67] Routine screening for zinc deficiency is recommended after gastric bypass, and routine supplementation is recommended following biliopancreatic diversion (with or without duodenal switch). Copper deficiency can present as anemia and neurologic impairment. For mild to moderate deficiency, 3 to 8 mg/d of calcium gluconate is recommended until copper levels come to normal and, in severe cases, 2 to 4 mg/d of intravenous copper for 6 days until the neurologic symptoms resolve and serum levels normalize.[54]

Pregnancy and Bariatric Surgery

At present, women of reproductive age (18–45 years) account for half of all bariatric surgery patients.[68] The American College of Obstetricians and Gynecologists recommends avoiding pregnancy for 12 to 24 months following bariatric surgery. During this time frame, many patients experience rapid weight loss and therefore are at risk for nutritional deficiencies.[69] However, some studies do not find any difference in neonatal outcomes based on the time interval between surgery and conception. The various bariatric procedures do not differentially affect outcomes of pregnancy.[70]

Relative to the general population, studies show that infants born after bariatric surgery are more likely to be premature and small for their gestational age.[71] Rates of cesarean section are not different between women who have and have not undergone bariatric surgery.[72] Women becoming pregnant after bariatric surgery are at risk for postoperative complications such as internal hernia, and the early involvement of a bariatric surgeon in such cases is recommended.[69]

SUMMARY

Bariatric surgery is the best known treatment of obesity. The sleeve gastrectomy and Roux-en-Y gastric bypass are the two most popular bariatric operations, and one cannot conclusively be considered superior to the other. Bariatric surgery has the potential to improve multiple obesity-related comorbidities, such as T2DM, cardiovascular disease, and sleep apnea. The effect of bariatric surgery on weight loss and comorbidities varies by the type of procedure.

REFERENCES

1. Flegal KM, Carroll MD, Kit BK, et al. Prevalence of obesity and trends in the distribution of body mass index among US adults, 1999-2010. JAMA 2012;307(5): 491-7.
2. Guh DP, Zhang W, Bansback N, et al. The incidence of co-morbidities related to obesity and overweight: a systematic review and meta-analysis. BMC Public Health 2009;9:88.
3. Danaei G, Ding EL, Mozaffarian D, et al. The preventable causes of death in the United States: comparative risk assessment of dietary, lifestyle, and metabolic risk factors. PLoS Med 2009;6(4):e1000058.
4. Lindekilde N, Gladstone BP, Lubeck M, et al. The impact of bariatric surgery on quality of life: a systematic review and meta-analysis. Obes Rev 2015;16(8): 639-51.
5. Maggard MA, Shugarman LR, Suttorp M, et al. Meta-analysis: surgical treatment of obesity. Ann Intern Med 2005;142(7):547-59.
6. Gloy VL, Briel M, Bhatt DL, et al. Bariatric surgery versus non-surgical treatment for obesity: a systematic review and meta-analysis of randomised controlled trials. BMJ 2013;347:f5934.
7. Nguyen NT, Vu S, Kim E, et al. Trends in utilization of bariatric surgery, 2009-2012. Surg Endosc 2015;30(7):2723-7.
8. International Federation for the Surgery of Obesity and Metabolic Disorders. Bariatric surgery. 2014. Available at: http://www.ifso.com/bariatric-surgery/. Accessed May 10, 2016.
9. Khwaja H, Coelho AJ, Mazzarella M, et al. The IFSO Website (http://www.ifso.com): the online gateway to obesity and metabolic disorders for bariatric surgery professionals and patients: on behalf of the IFSO Communications Committee. Obes Surg 2015;25(11):2176-9.
10. US Food and Drug Administration. Gastric banding. 2015. Available at: http://www.fda.gov/MedicalDevices/ProductsandMedicalProcedures/ObesityDevices/ucm350132.htm. Accessed May 10, 2016.
11. Scopinaro N, Gianetta E, Civalleri D, et al. Two years of clinical experience with biliopancreatic bypass for obesity. Am J Clin Nutr 1980;33(2 Suppl):506-14.
12. Hess DS, Hess DW. Biliopancreatic diversion with a duodenal switch. Obes Surg 1998;8(3):267-82.

13. Buchwald H, Oien DM. Metabolic/bariatric surgery worldwide 2011. Obes Surg 2013;23(4):427–36.
14. Ashrafian H, le Roux CW, Rowland SP, et al. Metabolic surgery and obstructive sleep apnoea: the protective effects of bariatric procedures. Thorax 2012; 67(5):442–9.
15. Chakravartty S, Tassinari D, Salerno A, et al. What is the mechanism behind weight loss maintenance with gastric bypass? Curr Obes Rep 2015;4(2):262–8.
16. Benaiges D, Mas-Lorenzo A, Goday A, et al. Laparoscopic sleeve gastrectomy: more than a restrictive bariatric surgery procedure? World J Gastroenterol 2015; 21(41):11804–14.
17. Himpens J, Cadiere GB, Bazi M, et al. Long-term outcomes of laparoscopic adjustable gastric banding. Arch Surg 2011;146(7):802–7.
18. Franco JV, Ruiz PA, Palermo M, et al. A review of studies comparing three laparoscopic procedures in bariatric surgery: sleeve gastrectomy, Roux-en-Y gastric bypass and adjustable gastric banding. Obes Surg 2011;21(9):1458–68.
19. Fischer L, Hildebrandt C, Bruckner T, et al. Excessive weight loss after sleeve gastrectomy: a systematic review. Obes Surg 2012;22(5):721–31.
20. Trastulli S, Desiderio J, Guarino S, et al. Laparoscopic sleeve gastrectomy compared with other bariatric surgical procedures: a systematic review of randomized trials. Surg Obes Relat Dis 2013;9(5):816–29.
21. Higa K, Ho T, Tercero F, et al. Laparoscopic Roux-en-Y gastric bypass: 10-year follow-up. Surg Obes Relat Dis 2011;7(4):516–25.
22. Carlin AM, Zeni TM, English WJ, et al. The comparative effectiveness of sleeve gastrectomy, gastric bypass, and adjustable gastric banding procedures for the treatment of morbid obesity. Ann Surg 2013;257(5):791–7.
23. Clough A, Hamill D, Jackson S, et al. Outcome of three common bariatric procedures in the public sector. ANZ J Surg 2016. [Epub ahead of print].
24. Li J, Lai D, Wu D. Laparoscopic Roux-en-Y gastric bypass versus laparoscopic sleeve gastrectomy to treat morbid obesity-related comorbidities: a systematic review and meta-analysis. Obes Surg 2016;26(2):429–42.
25. Zhang C, Yuan Y, Qiu C, et al. A meta-analysis of 2-year effect after surgery: laparoscopic Roux-en-Y gastric bypass versus laparoscopic sleeve gastrectomy for morbid obesity and diabetes mellitus. Obes Surg 2014;24(9):1528–35.
26. Dumon KR, Murayama KM. Bariatric surgery outcomes. Surg Clin North Am 2011;91(6):1313–38, x.
27. Kwok CS, Pradhan A, Khan MA, et al. Bariatric surgery and its impact on cardiovascular disease and mortality: a systematic review and meta-analysis. Int J Cardiol 2014;173(1):20–8.
28. Schauer DP, Arterburn DE, Livingston EH, et al. Impact of bariatric surgery on life expectancy in severely obese patients with diabetes: a decision analysis. Ann Surg 2015;261(5):914–9.
29. Amstutz S, Michel JM, Kopp S, et al. Potential benefits of prophylactic cholecystectomy in patients undergoing bariatric bypass surgery. Obes Surg 2015;25(11): 2054–60.
30. Tsirline VB, Keilani ZM, El Djouzi S, et al. How frequently and when do patients undergo cholecystectomy after bariatric surgery? Surg Obes Relat Dis 2014; 10(2):313–21.
31. Plecka Ostlund M, Wenger U, Mattsson F, et al. Population-based study of the need for cholecystectomy after obesity surgery. Br J Surg 2012;99(6):864–9.
32. Hannah WN Jr, Harrison SA. Effect of weight loss, diet, exercise, and bariatric surgery on nonalcoholic fatty liver disease. Clin Liver Dis 2016;20(2):339–50.

33. Bower G, Toma T, Harling L, et al. Bariatric surgery and non-alcoholic fatty liver disease: a systematic review of liver biochemistry and histology. Obes Surg 2015;25(12):2280–9.

34. Dent J, El-Serag HB, Wallander MA, et al. Epidemiology of gastro-oesophageal reflux disease: a systematic review. Gut 2005;54(5):710–7.

35. Oor JE, Roks DJ, Unlu C, et al. Laparoscopic sleeve gastrectomy and gastro-esophageal reflux disease: a systematic review and meta-analysis. Am J Surg 2016;211(1):250–67.

36. Pallati PK, Shaligram A, Shostrom VK, et al. Improvement in gastroesophageal reflux disease symptoms after various bariatric procedures: review of the bariatric outcomes longitudinal database. Surg Obes Relat Dis 2014;10(3):502–7.

37. de Jong JR, van Ramshorst B, Timmer R, et al. The influence of laparoscopic adjustable gastric banding on gastroesophageal reflux. Obes Surg 2004;14(3):399–406.

38. de Jong JR, Besselink MG, van Ramshorst B, et al. Effects of adjustable gastric banding on gastroesophageal reflux and esophageal motility: a systematic review. Obes Rev 2010;11(4):297–305.

39. Gutschow CA, Collet P, Prenzel K, et al. Long-term results and gastroesophageal reflux in a series of laparoscopic adjustable gastric banding. J Gastrointest Surg 2005;9(7):941–8.

40. Steed H, Walsh S, Reynolds N. A brief report of the epidemiology of obesity in the inflammatory bowel disease population of Tayside, Scotland. Obes Facts 2009; 2(6):370–2.

41. Keidar A, Hazan D, Sadot E, et al. The role of bariatric surgery in morbidly obese patients with inflammatory bowel disease. Surg Obes Relat Dis 2015;11(1):132–6.

42. Aminian A, Andalib A, Ver MR, et al. Outcomes of bariatric surgery in patients with inflammatory bowel disease. Obes Surg 2015;26(6):1186–90.

43. Schauer PR, Kashyap SR, Wolski K, et al. Bariatric surgery versus intensive medical therapy in obese patients with diabetes. N Engl J Med 2012;366(17):1567–76.

44. Maestro A, Rigla M, Caixas A. Does bariatric surgery reduce cancer risk? a review of the literature. Endocrinol Nutr 2015;62(3):138–43.

45. Mingrone G, Panunzi S, De Gaetano A, et al. Bariatric surgery versus conventional medical therapy for type 2 diabetes. N Engl J Med 2012;366(17):1577–85.

46. Schauer PR, Bhatt DL, Kirwan JP, et al. Bariatric surgery versus intensive medical therapy for diabetes–3-year outcomes. N Engl J Med 2014;370(21):2002–13.

47. Mingrone G, Panunzi S, De Gaetano A, et al. Bariatric-metabolic surgery versus conventional medical treatment in obese patients with type 2 diabetes: 5 year follow-up of an open-label, single-centre, randomised controlled trial. Lancet 2015;386(9997):964–73.

48. Robert M, Belanger P, Hould FS, et al. Should metabolic surgery be offered in morbidly obese patients with type I diabetes? Surg Obes Relat Dis 2015;11(4):798–805.

49. Ashrafian H, Toma T, Rowland SP, et al. Bariatric surgery or non-surgical weight loss for obstructive sleep apnoea? A systematic review and comparison of meta-analyses. Obes Surg 2015;25(7):1239–50.

50. Sarkhosh K, Switzer NJ, El-Hadi M, et al. The impact of bariatric surgery on obstructive sleep apnea: a systematic review. Obes Surg 2013;23(3):414–23.

51. Kaidar-Person O, Person B, Szomstein S, et al. Nutritional deficiencies in morbidly obese patients: a new form of malnutrition? Part A: vitamins. Obes Surg 2008; 18(7):870–6.

52. Kaidar-Person O, Person B, Szomstein S, et al. Nutritional deficiencies in morbidly obese patients: a new form of malnutrition? Part B: minerals. Obes Surg 2008; 18(8):1028–34.

53. Davies DJ, Baxter JM, Baxter JN. Nutritional deficiencies after bariatric surgery. Obes Surg 2007;17(9):1150–8.

54. Mechanick JI, Youdim A, Jones DB, et al. Clinical practice guidelines for the perioperative nutritional, metabolic, and nonsurgical support of the bariatric surgery patient–2013 update: cosponsored by American Association of Clinical Endocrinologists, the Obesity Society, and American Society for Metabolic & Bariatric Surgery. Obesity (Silver Spring) 2013;21(Suppl 1):S1–27.

55. Dolan K, Hatzifotis M, Newbury L, et al. A clinical and nutritional comparison of biliopancreatic diversion with and without duodenal switch. Ann Surg 2004; 240(1):51–6.

56. Ramirez Prada D, Delgado G, Hidalgo Patino CA, et al. Using of WHO guidelines for the management of severe malnutrition to cases of marasmus and kwashiorkor in a Colombia children's hospital. Nutr Hosp 2011;26(5):977–83.

57. Vargas-Ruiz AG, Hernandez-Rivera G, Herrera MF. Prevalence of iron, folate, and vitamin B12 deficiency anemia after laparoscopic Roux-en-Y gastric bypass. Obes Surg 2008;18(3):288–93.

58. Rabkin RA, Rabkin JM, Metcalf B, et al. Nutritional markers following duodenal switch for morbid obesity. Obes Surg 2004;14(1):84–90.

59. van Rutte PW, Aarts EO, Smulders JF, et al. Nutrient deficiencies before and after sleeve gastrectomy. Obes Surg 2014;24(10):1639–46.

60. Flancbaum L, Belsley S, Drake V, et al. Preoperative nutritional status of patients undergoing Roux-en-Y gastric bypass for morbid obesity. J Gastrointest Surg 2006;10(7):1033–7.

61. Koch TR, Finelli FC. Postoperative metabolic and nutritional complications of bariatric surgery. Gastroenterol Clin North Am 2010;39(1):109–24.

62. Handzlik-Orlik G, Holecki M, Orlik B, et al. Nutrition management of the postbariatric surgery patient. Nutr Clin Pract 2015;30(3):383–92.

63. Slater GH, Ren CJ, Siegel N, et al. Serum fat-soluble vitamin deficiency and abnormal calcium metabolism after malabsorptive bariatric surgery. J Gastrointest Surg 2004;8(1):48–55 [discussion: 54–5].

64. Karefylakis C, Naslund I, Edholm D, et al. Vitamin D status 10 years after primary gastric bypass: gravely high prevalence of hypovitaminosis D and raised PTH levels. Obes Surg 2014;24(3):343–8.

65. Aills L, Blankenship J, Buffington C, et al. ASMBS allied health nutritional guidelines for the surgical weight loss patient. Surg Obes Relat Dis 2008;4(5 Suppl): S73–108.

66. Saif T, Strain GW, Dakin G, et al. Evaluation of nutrient status after laparoscopic sleeve gastrectomy 1, 3, and 5 years after surgery. Surg Obes Relat Dis 2012; 8(5):542–7.

67. Isom KA, Andromalos L, Ariagno M, et al. Nutrition and metabolic support recommendations for the bariatric patient. Nutr Clin Pract 2014;29(6):718–39.

68. Shekelle PG, Newberry S, Maglione M, et al. Bariatric surgery in women of reproductive age: special concerns for pregnancy. Evid Rep Technol Assess (Full Rep) 2008;169:1–51.

69. American College of Obstetricians and Gynecologists. ACOG practice bulletin no. 105: bariatric surgery and pregnancy. Obstet Gynecol 2009;113(6):1405–13.
70. Ducarme G, Parisio L, Santulli P, et al. Neonatal outcomes in pregnancies after bariatric surgery: a retrospective multi-centric cohort study in three French referral centers. J Matern Fetal Neonatal Med 2013;26(3):275–8.
71. Johansson K, Cnattingius S, Naslund I, et al. Outcomes of pregnancy after bariatric surgery. N Engl J Med 2015;372(9):814–24.
72. Roos N, Neovius M, Cnattingius S, et al. Perinatal outcomes after bariatric surgery: nationwide population based matched cohort study. BMJ 2013;347:f6460.

Future Therapies in Obesity

Octavia Pickett-Blakely, MD, MHS[a],*, Carolyn Newberry, MD[b]

KEYWORDS

- Obesity • Pharmacotherapy • Endobariatrics • Genetics • Microbiome
- Complementary/alternative therapies

KEY POINTS

- Obesity involves multiple pathophysiologic processes that can be targets for treatment.
- Endobariatric procedures are effective weight loss therapies.
- Microbiome manipulation is a popular area of study that holds promise for the treatment of obesity.

INTRODUCTION

As outlined earlier in this issue, obesity has grown to epidemic proportions in the past 3 decades. However, there has been a major lag in the development of effective therapies for obesity. Although the obesity epidemic is largely explained by environmental factors, such as calorie-dense diets and sedentary lifestyles, the discovery of other contributing factors, such as altered intestinal microbiota and genetic derangement, has unlocked additional therapeutic pathways. Therefore, development of novel therapeutic interventions for obesity is in high demand and remains an active area of investigation. Although the mainstay of therapy is behavioral modifications via diet and exercise, innovative pharmaceutical, mechanical, hormonal, and device options are introduced in this article.

PHARMACOTHERAPY

There are numerous pharmacologic targets for the treatment of obesity. Pharmacotherapy for obesity is covered extensively (see Jeanette N. Keith's article, "Pharmacotherapy in Treatment of Obesity," in this issue), but this article discusses possible new therapies that may be used as a supplement to diet therapy and exercise.

[a] GI Nutrition, Obesity and Celiac Disease Program, Division of Gastroenterology, University of Pennsylvania Perelman School of Medicine, 3400 Convention Avenue, 4 South, Philadelphia, PA 19104, USA; [b] Division of Gastroenterology, University of Pennsylvania Perelman School of Medicine, Philadelphia, PA 19104, USA
* Corresponding author.
E-mail address: octavia.pickett-blakely@uphs.upenn.edu

Gastroenterol Clin N Am 45 (2016) 705–714
http://dx.doi.org/10.1016/j.gtc.2016.07.008
0889-8553/16/© 2016 Elsevier Inc. All rights reserved.

Therapeutic targets address 3 basic mechanisms: (1) decreasing caloric intake/absorption, (2) increasing energy expenditure, and (3) modulation of adipocytes. To date, most of the drugs approved for the treatment of obesity decrease oral intake by suppressing appetite via central nervous system neurotransmitters. However, other physiologic pathways hold promise as potential therapeutic targets.

Decrease Caloric Intake/Increase Energy Expenditure

Beloranib is a drug that inhibits methionine aminopeptidase 2, an enzyme involved in fat biosynthesis, oxidation, and breakdown. Caloric intake is also reportedly decreased in patients treated with beloranib and is associated with an increased level of serum adiponectin. Based on early data, beloranib seems to be an effective weight loss agent. In a 12-week, phase II trial, beloranib resulted in significantly greater weight loss compared with placebo (-10.9 ± 1.1 kg vs -0.4 ± 0.4 kg, respectively; $P < .0001$ vs placebo).[1] Compared with the currently available pharmacotherapies, beloranib may have a promising future in light of the robust weight loss observed in early studies.

Gut hormones have been heavily investigated as potential therapeutic interventions for obesity. As an endocrine organ, the gastrointestinal tract secretes numerous neurohormones that affect energy intake and satiety.[2,3] For example, amylin (synthetic analogue of Symlin) is a beta cell–derived peptide that slows gastric emptying and decreases food intake. Likewise, glucagonlike peptide 1(GLP-1) has similar physiologic effects and the synthetic GLP-1 agonist liraglutide (Saxenda) is US Food and Drug Administration (FDA) approved for weight loss.[2] Other neurohormones that also decrease food intake include pancreatic polypeptide, which is secreted from the pancreas; ghrelin, which is secreted from the stomach; oxyntomodulin and peptide YY, which are secreted from intestinal L cells; and cholecystokinin, which is secreted from the small bowel.[2,3] Given the many gut neurohormones involved in food intake, a combined pharmacologic approach targeting multiple physiologic pathways may offer optimal efficacy to treat obesity.

Adipocyte Modulation/Increase Energy Expenditure

Adipose tissue is metabolically active tissue and has been targeted as a potential therapeutic pathway for obesity. In particular, brown adipose tissue (BAT), which is less functional in obese versus lean individuals, is involved in fat burning and thermogenesis.[4] In contrast, white adipose tissue (WAT) is responsible for obesity. A recent animal study used nanoparticles that selectively delivered rosiglitazone (peroxisome proliferator-activated receptor gamma) and prostaglandin E2 to adipose tissue leading to (1) transformation of WAT to the thermogenic BAT, and (2) increased angiogenesis-induced expansion of BAT.[5] Increasing the conversion of WAT to thermogenic BAT is an attractive method to increase energy expenditure and ultimately weight loss. An recently proposed additional target for brown fat activation is mirabegron (Myrbetriq), which is a β3-adrenoceptor agonist currently used to treat overactive bladder. β3-Adrenoceptor agonism has been shown to increase resting the basal metabolic rate in humans,[6] but whether this increase leads to substantial weight loss remains to be seen.

ENDOBARIATRICS

Endoscopic bariatric therapies (EBTs) represent an evolving and exciting therapy for obesity. Discussed in detail elsewhere in this issue, EBTs offer an effective weight loss option for individuals who fail traditional therapies and/or are not eligible for (or do not wish to) undergo weight loss surgery. These procedures also may serve as bridge procedures for patients who are at high operative risk given their obesity.[7] These therapies are minimally invasive, well tolerated, and effective in achieving weight loss goals in the general population.[8] As of 2016, the 3 FDA-approved EBTs are the Orbera Intragastric Balloon, the Reshape Dual Balloon, and the Aspire Assist, with more devices and procedures expected to be approved in the coming years.

Space-occupying Devices

Reduction of intragastric capacitance through space-occupying devices is the physiologic basis for restrictive EBTs, such as the Orbera Intragastric Balloon and the Reshape Dual Balloon. In addition to the mechanical restriction, reduction in hunger may also lead to decreased energy intake.[9,10] Several other intragastric balloons are also currently being studied, including an adjustable saline-filled device called the Spatz Adjustable Balloon System, and gas-filled balloons that can be either orally ingested (Obalon Gastric Balloon, Ullorex) or endoscopically placed (Heliosphere). However, complications related to catheter migration, device rupture, and short-term efficacy have hindered their approval, with more studies being conducted to alter these devices to bring them safely to market.[11–13]

The Transpyloric Shuttle is a bispherical device with smaller and larger bulbs that are deployed endoscopically through an overtube, resting within the gastric antrum and traversing the pylorus to delay gastric emptying and induce early satiety.[14] It is currently undergoing a multicenter trial in the United States after preliminary data showed positive feasibility and safety profiles.[15]

Gastroplasty

Traditionally, gastroplasty is a surgical procedure; however, with the advent of several new FDA-approved devices, this can now be achieved endoscopically. One method is the primary obesity surgery endoluminal procedure, which uses full-thickness tissue plication within the gastric fundus and distal body to limit gastric accommodation, delay gastric emptying, and promote early satiety.[16] Endoluminal vertical gastroplasty is an alternative option, using suture or staple placement along the greater curvature of the stomach and producing results similar to a traditional gastric sleeve.[17] These procedures remain under investigation in the United States, but have shown promising results in early studies.[14]

Aspiration Therapy

Aspiration therapy is a method of weight loss that results from the disposal of approximately one-third of the gastric contents after each meal. The gastric contents are eliminated through the use of a specially formulated gastrostomy tube with a one-way valve known as the AspireAssist.[8] The AspireAssist device was recently approved by the FDA after its efficacy was proved in the domestic and international literature with high excess weight loss at 6 months and low complications in patients with a broad body mass index range of 35 to 55 kg/m^2.[18,19]

OTHER MODALITIES
Gastric Electric Stimulation

Although not a novel concept, gastric electric stimulation is a modality on the therapeutic horizon for the management of obesity. The rationale for gastric electric stimulation involves exerting control over vagal nerve–induced secretion of neuropeptides that signal satiety in the central nervous system.[20,21] Since its inception more than a decade ago, there have been numerous iterations of the devices integrating this concept. One such device is the MAESTRO/Vbloc system, which also includes vagal nerve blockade. In addition to neurohormones (eg, GLP-1 and cholecystokinin), the vagus nerve is highly involved in energy intake.[22] Among other factors, gastric distension induces satiety via vagal nerve afferent signals. Given the relation of the vagus nerve to energy metabolism, it is a worthy target as an obesity therapy. Early studies of the Vbloc system showed unimpressive weight loss with only small differences compared with placebo.[23] More recently, a double-blind placebo-controlled study by Morton and colleagues[22] showed significantly greater weight loss in subjects in the treatment group (11% total weight loss) compared with the sham group (6% total weight loss). Through continued research, it is hoped that this product will be added to the therapeutic arsenal in the future.

Gene Therapy

Although environmental factors account for most obesity cases, genetic alterations of single, and in some cases multiple, genes result in the predisposition to and development of obesity. To date, hundreds of obesity-linked genes have been identified.[24] Although a detailed review is beyond the scope of this article, some of the significant genes and their potential therapeutic impacts are highlighted.

To date, one of the most notable models of genetically linked obesity is the leptin-deficient ob/ob mouse model. Leptin is a multifunction neurohormone secreted by WAT that acts in the hypothalamic region of the brain to regulate food intake.[25] The leptin-deficient ob/ob mouse develops obesity in the setting of excessive caloric intake.[25] In addition, a leptin receptor gene defect has also been shown in animal models and humans to cause early-onset obesity.[25] In contrast with the leptin-deficient model, in the setting of a leptin receptor gene defect, administration of leptin does not reverse obesity. Pro-opiomelanocortin (POMC) is also involved in the regulation of food intake.[26] Its action is partially mediated via melanocyte-stimulating hormone and adrenocorticotrophic hormone and it is deficient in obese individuals.[26] Individual patients with impaired POMC function developed early-onset obesity, adrenal insufficiency, and red hair pigmentation.[27] Uncoupling proteins (UCPs) are a group of proteins involved in thermogenesis and several defective UCP genes have been associated with weight gain in adulthood.[28] Furthermore, given that the process of thermogenesis is under autonomic nervous system control, knockout models with defective adrenergic receptors showed an increased propensity toward obesity with ingestion of a high-fat diet.[28] The aforementioned genes are only a few of many that may serve as potential candidates for therapeutic gene therapy. In particular, treatment of the leptin-deficient ob/ob mouse with leptin delivered via an adenovirus vector resulted in significant weight loss. Using the data from observations in the ob/ob mouse model, humans treated with physiologic doses of recombinant leptin therapy have shown successful weight loss.[29] There are also polygenic and syndromic forms of obesity that result from multiple genetic defects and/or chromosomal abnormalities.[24] Gene therapy may prove more challenging in these patients given the multiple defects that result in the obesity phenotype.

Intestinal Microbiome Manipulation

The gut microbiome has been implicated as a potential contributor to the obesity epidemic following several observations in animal models. Backhead and colleagues[30,31] showed that gut microbes are involved in the regulation of fat storage, energy harvest, glucose intestinal absorption, short-chain fatty acid (SCFA) fermentation, and triglyceride synthesis. There are also epidemiologic data linking antibiotic exposure in the perinatal period and infancy to altered gut flora and childhood obesity, respectively.[32] Thus, manipulation of the intestinal microbiome has been proposed as a prospective therapeutic target for obesity. Alteration of the microbiome may be achieved via a variety of methods like diet/diet supplements, and the use of prebiotics and probiotics.

Prebiotics are oligosaccharides that bypass intestinal absorption and are in turn fermented by colonic microbes to produce SCFAs.[33] SCFAs may be used by colonocytes as fuel and also alter the intestinal flora. Intestinal bifidobacteria, a species that has been associated with a favorable metabolic profile, are increased with prebiotic use.[34] Furthermore, prebiotic ingestion in rats causes increased peptide YY and GLP-1 and decreased gastric emptying and food intake.[35] When examined in a randomized control trial, oligofructose supplementation resulted in a small but significant proportion of weight loss compared with weight gain in the placebo group.[36] The observed weight loss was associated with decreased ghrelin and increased peptide YY levels as well.[36] More recently, a prebiotic formulation selectively delivered to the colon was shown to reduce weight gain, intra-abdominal adipose tissue distribution, and hepatic fat, and prevented progression of insulin sensitivity.[37] In the Fat-1 mouse model of antibiotic-induced obesity, omega-3 fatty acid supplementation decreases antibiotic-induced obesity. This mouse makes endogenous n-3 polyunsaturated fatty acids (PUFAs) from n-6 PUFAs and ultimately leads to a reduced Firmicutes/Bacteroidetes ratio and bifidobacteria/Enterobacteriaceae ratio as well as inflammatory markers such as tumor necrosis factor alpha and interleukin 6.[38]

Probiotics are microorganisms that provide a health benefit to the host. The obesity phenotype is associated with altered microbial profiles; for example, decreased Bifidobacterium and increased Firmicutes species. Altered gut microbiota results in greater energy harvest with subsequent weight gain and increased body fat in mouse models.[39,40] Furthermore, a lesser degree of gut microbiota richness is linked to increased adiposity, insulin resistance, and dyslipidemia in humans.[41] Hence, it is possible that supplementation with favorable bacteria may tip the scales in the direction of a nonobese phenotype, whereas antibiotics that diminish the favorable bacterial profile may promote an obese phenotype. Although the data are mixed, there are several studies that suggest that probiotic supplementation is associated with weight loss and an improved metabolic profile.[42] One of the largest and longest studies (6 months) evaluating the effect of supplemental probiotics (in addition to a calorie-restricted diet) showed no significant difference in weight in the treatment and placebo groups. However, in women, there was significantly greater weight loss in the group receiving probiotic supplementation compared with the placebo group despite equal amounts of calorie restriction.[42]

Fecal microbiota transplant is the quintessential modality to manipulate the intestinal microbiota. In this procedure, the recipient's intestinal tract is populated with the fecal material from a healthy donor. This method has been used to restore the intestinal flora after recurrent *Clostridium difficile* infection with success and may be a promising option in the future for obesity.[43] Thus far, data in this area are limited; however, fecal microbiota transplant from lean donors to obese recipients has been shown to improve insulin sensitivity.[44]

Bioengineering/Biomaterial

As mentioned previously, BAT is an important contributor to thermogenesis and an obvious potential therapeutic target for obesity, whether by genetically modulated upregulation of uncoupling protein synthesis or pharmacologic expansion of uncoupling protein-positive BAT.[45] Transplant of biologically active BAT has been investigated in mouse models but tissue transplant bears the risk of graft-versus-host immunologic reactions.[45] As a result, alternative techniques have been investigated. Specifically, Tharp and colleagues[46] reported a novel method of transplanting BAT-like cells via a process called matrix-associated transplant. This method involves isolating stem cells from adipose tissue, differentiating them into beige adipose tissue cells, and then delivering them via a hyaluronic acid hydrogel matrix.[46] Mice that received the transplanted beige adipose tissue showed improved metabolic profiles compared with their WAT-transplanted mice counterparts, including lower resting glucose levels, lower serum triglyceride levels, and less weight gain when fed a 60% fat diet.[46]

Gelesis100 is a novel intervention consisting of a capsule filled with a biocompatible hydrogel that expands in the stomach after absorbing water. The expanded material results in increased intragastric volume and ultimately early satiety. The Gelesis100 material also acts as a barrier to glucose absorption in the small intestine. Similar to bariatric surgery, this product provides restrictive, maldigestive, and malabsorptive mechanisms to induce weight loss. Gelesis100 is currently under study, but is not yet FDA approved. However, early data have shown that a significantly greater proportion of overweight/obese subjects in the low-dose treatment arm lost 10% of their baseline body weight compared with placebo. The adverse effects were similar in both groups.[47] It remains to be seen whether Gelesis100 will prove to be an effective, minimally invasive supplemental therapy to standard behavioral modifications for obese individuals.

Complementary and Alternative Medicine

Complementary and alternative medicine (CAM) is a growing trend in recent years, augmenting traditional Western practices for the treatment of a variety of diseases, including obesity. Although not generally recommended as a sole therapy, CAM for weight loss has become increasingly popular as a way to take a more natural approach to healthy eating habits and lifestyle modifications through mediums such as hypnosis, mindfulness-based practices, acupuncture, and dietary supplements. Some of the available CAM therapies for obesity are listed in **Table 1**.

Originally gaining popularity in the medical community as an aid for smoking cessation, hypnosis is now being considered as an option for weight loss. Defined as the induction of a trancelike state that allows the use of therapeutic suggestion, hypnosis can be used in conjunction with cognitive behavior therapy to reduce stress-induced eating and increase awareness of healthy habits.[48] The data regarding the role of hypnosis in obesity treatment are conflicting, although there is some support for this modality to induce meaningful reduction in stress levels and subsequent calorie consumption.[49,50] In contrast with hypnosis, mindfulness-based practice allows behavioral modulation through the distancing of the patient from habitual thoughts, emotions, and behaviors to allow an enhanced presence and heightened adaptive responses. This treatment can be used to help guide decisions regarding calorie consumption and energy expenditure. Mindful-based practices include yoga, meditation, cognitive therapy, and eating awareness training. Although these modalities are popular for stress reduction, the literature shows minimal effect on weight loss efforts.[51]

Acupuncture involves the insertion of several fine needles into strategic positions in the body and has been used to treat a variety of medical conditions, including pain and stress. More recently acupuncture has been studied as an adjunctive therapy for weight loss. Hypothesized to alter neurotransmitter levels associated with satiety and appetite, including tyrosine, tryptophan, and dopamine, acupuncture has not consistently shown a beneficial effect with respect to weight loss in humans.[52]

Dietary supplements remain popular because of their wide availability and general tolerance despite a lack of data proving their effectiveness. The mechanisms of action of dietary supplements vary widely and include reducing caloric intake, inhibiting caloric absorption, increasing energy consumption, and preventing fat synthesis.[53] For example, conjugated linoleic acid, a mixture of linoleic acid isomers, alters body

Table 1
Summary of complementary and alternative therapies for obesity

Complementary and Alternative Therapies for Obesity			
Type of Intervention	Description	Proposed Mechanism	Application
Hypnotherapy	Induction of a trancelike state that enables the use of therapeutic suggestion	Used to encourage healthy diet and exercise habits and reduce stress-induced eating through regulated therapy sessions	Often used in conjunction with formalized cognitive behavioral therapy
Acupuncture	Ancient Chinese art of strategic positioning of fine needles along pressure points located throughout the body	Thought to alter neurotransmitter signals associated with satiety and appetite as well as reduce overall stress levels	Can be used alone or in combination with other alternative-based practices
Mindfulness-based practice	Awareness training designed to distance the patient from habitual thoughts and behaviors to enhance presence and adaptive responses to the environment	Used as a stress reducer and allows the practicer to experience a heightened awareness of healthy lifestyle choices	Conducted through several modalities, including yoga, meditation, and eating awareness training
Dietary supplements	Ingestible products that contain dietary ingredients, including vitamins, minerals, and amino acids, that are intended to add nutritional value to a standard diet	Multiple proposed mechanisms, including appetite suppression, nutrient absorption inhibition, metabolic stimulation, and fat synthesis suppression	Orally ingested in combination with a healthy diet

composition by reducing fat and increasing muscle mass in mice but human studies are less convincing.[54] Citrus aurantium (also known as bitter orange), is derived from the orange fruit tree and contains synephrine, an adrenergic agonist that stimulates metabolism. Although modest weight loss has been observed with consistent use, the safety profile is questionable given cardiovascular and cerebrovascular complications.[55] Garcinia cambogia is derived from a fruit-bearing plant native to southeastern Asia, and has received recent attention for its ability to suppress de novo fatty acid synthesis by inhibition of extramitochondrial citrate lysis. Despite its popularity and promising data from animal studies, significant weight loss in humans was not shown in a recent meta-analysis.[56]

SUMMARY

Obesity is a multifaceted disease that requires a treatment approach that considers all of the pathologic processes involved. Although behavioral modifications through diet and exercise are the mainstay of therapy for obesity, as a single approach, efficacy is limited and supplemental therapies are needed. The potential therapies discussed here range from hypnosis to intragastric space-occupying devices that hinder food intake. All therapies should ultimately result in decreased energy intake, increased energy expenditure, and/or decreased lipogenesis in order to enhance the therapeutic armamentarium for obesity.

REFERENCES

1. Kim DD, Krishnarajah J, Lillioja S, et al. Efficacy and safety of beloranib for weight loss in obese adults: a randomized controlled trial. Diabetes Obes Metab 2015; 17(6):566–72.
2. Davenport RJ, Wright S. Treating obesity: is it all in the gut? Drug Discov Today 2014;19(7):845–58.
3. Choudhury SM, Tan TM, Bloom SR. Gastrointestinal hormones and their role in obesity. Curr Opin Endocrinol Diabetes Obes 2016;23(1):18–22.
4. Honek J, Lim S, Fischer C, et al. Brown adipose tissue, thermogenesis, angiogenesis: pathophysiological aspects. Horm Mol Biol Clin Investig 2014;19(1):5–11.
5. Xue Y, Xu X, Zhang XQ, et al. Preventing diet-induced obesity in mice by adipose tissue transformation and angiogenesis using targeted nanoparticles. Proc Natl Acad Sci U S A 2016;113(20):5552–7.
6. Cypess AM, Weiner LS, Roberts-Toler C, et al. Activation of human brown adipose tissue by a beta3-adrenergic receptor agonist. Cell Metab 2015;21(1):33–8.
7. Zerrweck C, Maunoury V, Caiazzo R, et al. Preoperative weight loss with intragastric balloon decreases the risk of significant adverse outcomes of laparoscopic gastric bypass in super-super obese patients. Obes Surg 2012;22(5):777–82.
8. Goyal D, Watson RR. Endoscopic bariatric therapies. Curr Gastroenterol Rep 2016;18(6):26.
9. Konopko-Zubrzycka M, Baniukiewicz A, Wróblewski E, et al. The effect of intragastric balloon on plasma ghrelin, leptin, and adiponectin levels in patients with morbid obesity. J Clin Endocrinol Metab 2009;94(5):1644–9.
10. Kotzampassi K, Grosomanidis V, Papakostas P, et al. 500 intragastric balloons: what happens 5 years thereafter? Obes Surg 2012;22(6):896–903.
11. Machytka E, Klvana P, Kornbluth A, et al. Adjustable intragastric balloons: a 12-month pilot trial in endoscopic weight loss management. Obes Surg 2011;21(10): 1499–507.
12. Mion F, Ibrahim M, Marjoux S, et al. Swallowable Obalon(R) gastric balloons as an aid for weight loss: a pilot feasibility study. Obes Surg 2013;23(5):730–3.
13. Štimac D, Klobučar Majanović S, Ličina M. Recent trends in endoscopic management of obesity. Surg Innov 2016. [Epub ahead of print].
14. Sampath K, Dinani AM, Rothstein RI. Endoscopic devices for obesity. Curr Obes Rep 2016;5(2):251–61.
15. Marinos G, Eliades C, Raman Muthusamy V, et al. Weight loss and improved quality of life with a nonsurgical endoscopic treatment for obesity: clinical results from a 3- and 6-month study. Surg Obes Relat Dis 2014;10(5):929–34.
16. Lopez-Nava G, Bautista-Castano I, Jimenez A, et al. The primary obesity surgery endolumenal (POSE) procedure: one-year patient weight loss and safety outcomes. Surg Obes Relat Dis 2015;11(4):861–5.
17. Abu Dayyeh BK, Acosta A, Camilleri M, et al. Endoscopic sleeve gastroplasty alters gastric physiology and induces loss of body weight in obese individuals. Clin Gastroenterol Hepatol 2015. [Epub ahead of print].

18. Sullivan S, Stein R, Jonnalagadda S, et al. Aspiration therapy leads to weight loss in obese subjects: a pilot study. Gastroenterology 2013;145(6):1245–52.e1-5.
19. Forssell H, Noren E. A novel endoscopic weight loss therapy using gastric aspiration: results after 6 months. Endoscopy 2015;47(1):68–71.
20. Cha R, Marescaux J, Diana M. Updates on gastric electrical stimulation to treat obesity: systematic review and future perspectives. World J Gastrointest Endosc 2014;6(9):419–31.
21. Chiu JD, Soffer E. Gastric electrical stimulation for obesity. Curr Gastroenterol Rep 2015;17(1):424.
22. Morton GJ, Meek TH, Schwartz MW. Neurobiology of food intake in health and disease. Nat Rev Neurosci 2014;15(6):367–78.
23. Sarr MG, Billington CJ, Brancatisano R, et al. The EMPOWER study: randomized, prospective, double-blind, multicenter trial of vagal blockade to induce weight loss in morbid obesity. Obes Surg 2012;22(11):1771–82.
24. Gao M, Liu D. Gene therapy for obesity: progress and prospects. Discov Med 2014;17(96):319–28.
25. Zhang Y, Proenca R, Maffei M, et al. Positional cloning of the mouse obese gene and its human homologue. Nature 1994;372(6505):425–32.
26. Krude H, Biebermann H, Luck W, et al. Severe early-onset obesity, adrenal insufficiency and red hair pigmentation caused by POMC mutations in humans. Nat Genet 1998;19(2):155–7.
27. Farooqi IS, O'Rahilly S. Monogenic obesity in humans. Annu Rev Med 2005;56:443–58.
28. Ueta CB, Fernandes GW, Capelo LP, et al. Beta(1) adrenergic receptor is key to cold- and diet-induced thermogenesis in mice. J Endocrinol 2012;214(3):359–65.
29. Paz-Filho G, Wong ML, Licinio J. Ten years of leptin replacement therapy. Obes Rev 2011;12(5):e315–23.
30. Backhed F, Ley RE, Sonnenburg JL, et al. Host-bacterial mutualism in the human intestine. Science 2005;307(5717):1915–20.
31. Backhed F, Manchester JK, Semenkovich CF, et al. Mechanisms underlying the resistance to diet-induced obesity in germ-free mice. Proc Natl Acad Sci U S A 2007;104(3):979–84.
32. Turta O, Rautava S. Antibiotics, obesity and the link to microbes - what are we doing to our children? BMC Med 2016;14(1):57.
33. Patel R, DuPont HL. New approaches for bacteriotherapy: prebiotics, new-generation probiotics, and synbiotics. Clin Infect Dis 2015;60(Suppl 2):S108–21.
34. Bouhnik Y, Flourie B, D'Agay-Abensour L, et al. Administration of transgalacto-oligosaccharides increases fecal bifidobacteria and modifies colonic fermentation metabolism in healthy humans. J Nutr 1997;127(3):444–8.
35. Chambers ES, Morrison DJ, Frost G. Control of appetite and energy intake by SCFA: what are the potential underlying mechanisms? Proc Nutr Soc 2015;74(3):328–36.
36. Parnell JA, Reimer RA. Weight loss during oligofructose supplementation is associated with decreased ghrelin and increased peptide YY in overweight and obese adults. Am J Clin Nutr 2009;89(6):1751–9.
37. Chambers ES, Viardot A, Psichas A, et al. Effects of targeted delivery of propionate to the human colon on appetite regulation, body weight maintenance and adiposity in overweight adults. Gut 2015;64(11):1744–54.
38. Kaliannan K, Wang B, Li XY, et al. Omega-3 fatty acids prevent early-life antibiotic exposure-induced gut microbiota dysbiosis and later-life obesity. Int J Obes (Lond) 2016;40:1039–42.

39. Turnbaugh PJ, Ley RE, Mahowald MA, et al. An obesity-associated gut micro-biome with increased capacity for energy harvest. Nature 2006;444(7122): 1027–31.

40. Flint HJ. Obesity and the gut microbiota. J Clin Gastroenterol 2011;45(Suppl): S128–32.

41. Cotillard A, Kennedy SP, Kong LC, et al. Dietary intervention impact on gut micro-bial gene richness. Nature 2013;500(7464):585–8.

42. Saez-Lara MJ, Robles-Sanchez C, Ruiz-Ojeda FJ, et al. Effects of probiotics and synbiotics on obesity, insulin resistance syndrome, type 2 diabetes and non-alcoholic fatty liver disease: a review of human clinical trials. Int J Mol Sci 2016;17(6). http://dx.doi.org/10.3390/ijms17060928.

43. Ejtahed HS, Soroush AR, Angoorani P, et al. Gut microbiota as a target in the pathogenesis of metabolic disorders: a new approach to novel therapeutic agents. Horm Metab Res 2016;48(6):349–58.

44. Vrieze A, Van Nood E, Holleman F, et al. Transfer of intestinal microbiota from lean donors increases insulin sensitivity in individuals with metabolic syndrome. Gastroenterology 2012;143(4):913–6.e7.

45. Giralt M, Villarroya F. White, brown, beige/brite: different adipose cells for different functions? Endocrinology 2013;154(9):2992–3000.

46. Tharp KM, Jha AK, Kraiczy J, et al. Matrix-assisted transplantation of functional beige adipose tissue. Diabetes 2015;64(11):3713–24.

47. Astrup A, Kristensen M, Gness L, et al. Oral administration of Gelesis100, A novel hydrogel, significantly decreases body weight in overweight and obese subjects. Poster ICE/ENDO 20014 Meeting. Chicago, 2014.

48. Allison DB, Downey M, Atkinson RL, et al. Obesity as a disease: a white paper on evidence and arguments commissioned by the council of the obesity society. Obesity (Silver Spring) 2008;16(6):1161–77.

49. Kirsch I, Montgomery G, Sapirstein G. Hypnosis as an adjunct to cognitive-behavioral psychotherapy: a meta-analysis. J Consult Clin Psychol 1995;63(2): 214–20.

50. Stradling J, Roberts D, Wilson A, et al. Controlled trial of hypnotherapy for weight loss in patients with obstructive sleep apnoea. Int J Obes Relat Metab Disord 1998;22(3):278–81.

51. Daubenmier J, Kristeller J, Hecht FM, et al. Mindfulness intervention for stress eating to reduce cortisol and abdominal fat among overweight and obese women: an exploratory randomized controlled study. J Obes 2011;2011:651936.

52. Cho SH, Lee JS, Thabane L, et al. Acupuncture for obesity: a systematic review and meta-analysis. Int J Obes (Lond) 2009;33(2):183–96.

53. Pittler MH, Ernst E. Dietary supplements for body-weight reduction: a systematic review. Am J Clin Nutr 2004;79(4):529–36.

54. Silveira MB, Carraro R, Monereo S, et al. Conjugated linoleic acid (CLA) and obesity. Public Health Nutr 2007;10(10A):1181–6.

55. Haaz S, Fontaine KR, Cutter G, et al. Citrus aurantium and synephrine alkaloids in the treatment of overweight and obesity: an update. Obes Rev 2006;7(1):79–88.

56. Fassina P, Scherer Adami F, Terezinha Zani V, et al. The effect of garcinia cambo-gia as coadjuvant in the weight loss process. Nutr Hosp 2015;32(6):2400–8.

Childhood Overweight and Obesity

Jamilah Grant-Guimaraes, MD*, Ronald Feinstein, MD, Erica Laber, MD,
Jennifer Kosoy, MD

KEYWORDS

- Childhood • Overweight • Obesity • Comorbidity • Prevention • Assessment
- Treatment • Cultural

KEY POINTS

- Childhood overweight and obesity are increasing in prevalence and are a growing health concern.
- The diseases and their comorbidities have devastating consequences to children and adults as well as families, communities, and the nation. Comorbidities are cardiorespiratory, endocrinologic, gastrointestinal, orthopedic, and psychosocial.
- Health care providers are facing this crisis with limited medical, community, and federal resources and insufficient reimbursement.
- This article reviews recent trends in the assessment and treatment of this disease as well as trends in reimbursement, financial implications, and the need for further research and advocacy.

INTRODUCTION

According to the latest statistics from the Centers for Disease Control and Prevention, more than one-third (34.9% or 78.6 million) of US adults are obese, with an estimated annual medical cost of $147 billion in 2008. The prevalence of obesity in children increased 300% over approximately the past 40 years.[1] The National Health and Nutrition Examination Survey, 2009 to 2010, found 32% of children, 2 to 19 years old, to be overweight or obese, with 17% in the obese range. Children's risk varies significantly by race/ethnicity. In 2009 to 2010, 24% of non-Hispanic black, 21% of Hispanic, and greater than 20% of American Indian/Alaskan Native children and adolescents were obese compared with 14% of white children.[2] For children and adolescents aged 2 to 19 years, the prevalence of obesity has remained fairly stable at approximately 17% and affects approximately 12.7 million children and adolescents for the past decade; however, the prevalence of severe obesity in children continues to rise.[3]

Hofstra Northwell School of Medicine, Cohen Children's Medical Center, 269-01, 76th Avenue, New Hyde Park, NY 11040, USA
* Corresponding author.
E-mail address: jamarialia@gmail.com

Gastroenterol Clin N Am 45 (2016) 715–728
http://dx.doi.org/10.1016/j.gtc.2016.07.007
0889-8553/16/© 2016 Elsevier Inc. All rights reserved.

gastro.theclinics.com

Childhood overweight and obesity and their comorbidities threaten to prevent a significant portion of US children and adolescents from reaching their full potential and contributing to society on personal and community levels. Comorbidities of pediatric overweight and obesity are cardiovascular, endocrinologic, orthopedic, gastrointestinal, neurologic, pulmonary, and psychosocial (**Table 1**).[4,7,12,13] Children of underrepresented ethnic minority groups and those living at or below the poverty level are at increased risk. Communities of lower socioeconomic levels are burdened with obstacles concerning physical activity.[14,15] Children of parents with lower education levels, who are more likely to live in low-income/high-crime neighborhoods, are at increased risk for overweight and obesity.[16] School districts in these communities are less likely to have adequate funding to maintain physical education programs. Also, gym and recess are less likely to be supported during efforts to improve academic outcomes in failing schools.

Parents in low-income neighborhoods with high crime rates may be reluctant to allow children to play outside of the home. Both parents may be required to work, or single parents may need to work long hours to make ends meet, limiting their ability to eat together with their children and supervise food choices. Families living in food deserts face limitations in access to healthy foods, relying heavily on small community grocery stores or bodegas, where healthy choices are few and prices are high. Fast food restaurants are more prevalent in these communities, with the price of unhealthy fast food meals much less than that of local fruits and vegetables. Also, parents living in poverty are more likely to choose calorie-rich foods high in fat and simple carbohydrates and low in nutritional value, which they may consider more filling and more likely to maintain their children's satiety until the next meal can be obtained.

Pediatricians and other health care providers to children are faced with the daunting task of addressing this epidemic. They must identify those children and adolescents who are, or are at risk for becoming, overweight or obese, in addition to preventing the chronic illness of obesity in all children and adolescents and identifying those at increased risk. Primary care providers must accomplish this in the face of growing demands for relative value units, shrinking ancillary services and other support systems (such as social workers and nutritionists), decreasing or absent insurance reimbursement for obesity-related office visits, and unreasonably short time slots for patients.

This article has been written in an effort to provide necessary information and tools to health providers in dealing with the health crises of childhood overweight and obesity in the face of prevailing obstacles and limitations in medical practice. The pathophysiology, current theories, and trends in treatment, such as motivational interviewing, research, politics and policy, and specific needs for advocacy, are reviewed.

OVERVIEW

Obesity and its major comorbidities have become a major global health challenge affecting children and adolescents of all ages. The hope of ending its affects is through early identification and management, which are facilitated by the recognition of risk factors.

In addition to the socioeconomic factors discussed previously, epidemiologic and animal studies suggest potential links between intrauterine and postnatal factors and childhood obesity. Among these are the following.[17–20]

Intrauterine

- Maternal diabetes mellitus (gestational or type 1)
- Maternal hypertension
- Maternal gestational weight gain

Table 1
Comorbidities of childhood obesity

Cardiovascular	• Hyperlipidemia • Hypertension • Vascular dysfunction • Early coronary and aortic atherosclerosis[4] • Left ventricular and atrial enlargement and dysfunction[4]	The overall prevalence of dyslipidemia in the pediatric population has been reported as 20.3%, whereas that in overweight children is reported to be 42.9%.[5] The prevalence of clinically identified hypertension in United States children (estimates: prehypertension — 10%; hypertension — 3.7%) is directly correlated with increasing waist-circumference and BMI.[6] In a study by Gidding et al,[7] 48 children, 8–17 years old, with BMI of at least 40 kg/m^2 (obese by adult BMI measures) were studied using a graded stationary bicycle test. The subjects were noted to have deconditioning consistent with congestive heart failure.
Endocrinologic	• Metabolic syndrome • Hyperinsulinemia • Insulin resistance • Prediabetes • Type 2 diabetes mellitus	The prevalence of metabolic syndrome among pediatric patients, according to a systematic review of population-based studies, is 3.3% in nonobese, 11.9% in overweight, and 29.2% of obese children.[8] In another study, 50% of severely obese subjects had metabolic syndrome, whereas none of the normal-weight or overweight subjects did.[4] Up to 25% of severely obese adolescents are noted to have impaired glucose tolerance. The prevalence of pediatric type 2 diabetes mellitus is increased with obesity (one US sample noted a prevalence of 0.24/1000), and increases with age.[9,10]
Respiratory	Obstructive sleep apnea has been associated with childhood obesity.	Noted in 5.7%–36% of obese children and adolescents, this exceeds that noted in normal-weight children and adolescents, where the prevalence is estimated at 2%–3%.[4]
Gastrointestinal	• NASH • Cirrhosis • Liver failure requiring transplant	One study of adolescents with mean BMI of 59 kg/m^2 undergoing gastric bypass surgery noted liver involvement as follows[4]: 83% — nonalcoholic fatty liver disease 24% — steatosis 7% — fibrosis with steatosis 32% — inflammation with steatosis 20% — NASH

(continued on next page)

Table 1 (continued)		
Musculoskeletal	• Lower extremity arthralgias • Impaired mobility • Tibial bowing • Slipped capital femoral epiphysis	More than 80% of the children diagnosed with slipped capital femoral epiphysis are reportedly obese (BMI greater than the 95th percentile).[11]
Psychosocial	• Body image disturbances • Low self-esteem • Impaired socialization • Victimization • Depressive symptoms • Disordered eating • Anxiety	One study found that obesity in 10- and 11-year-old children independently predicted self-esteem 2 and 4 y later; obese children were 1.8 times more likely than normal-weight children to report low self-esteem at 4 y.[12]
Adult Obesity	Cumulative exposure to the risk factors for cardiovascular insults and the other components of the metabolic syndrome.	The Bogalusa Heart Study, a longitudinal analysis of children and later those same children as adults, helps demonstrate the risk of high BMI tracking into adulthood. Of the 26 children in 1 component of the study with BMI greater than the 99th percentile, 88% of those had an adult BMI of at least 35 kg/m², and 65% had an adult BMI of at least 40 kg/m².[13]

- Fetal growth (small for gestational age and large for gestational age)
- Fetal exposure to tobacco and cocaine

Postnatal

- Early introduction of solid foods (before age 4 months)
- Delayed weaning from bottles
- Breastfeeding less than 6 months
- Low strength of maternal-child relationship
- Increased screen time
- Parental obesity

Parental and family history of obesity may be linked to childhood obesity through genetic as well as environmental variables. Evidence for a significant role of gene-environment interactions has been demonstrated, where a genetic profile influences the ability to deal with the obesogenic impact of some environmental factors.[21] Children with obese parents and family members are likely to share similar patterns of diet, screen time, and physical activity and to be influenced by perspectives and attitudes concerning diet and activity that lead to overweight and obesity.

Studies have also suggested a link between changes of the microbiome (bacteria in the gut, which influence the processing of nutrients as well as immune and inflammatory responses) and the development of childhood obesity. Changes of this microbiome caused by perinatal antibiotic exposure seem to program the host to an obesity-prone metabolic phenotype, which persists even after the discontinuance of antibiotics and the recovery of the native gut flora. These changes may also be induced by the method of delivery (vaginal vs cesarean section) and antibiotic use during the first 2 years after birth.[17,22–24]

Definition and Identification

Obesity is most purely defined as excess fat. The manner in which a clinician identifies obesity usually relies on anthropometric measurements, such as height and weight. Other methods, such as underwater weighing (densitometry), multifrequency bioelectrical impedance analysis, and MRI used in research studies, are not practical in an office-based setting, where methods, such as body mass index (BMI) and measurements of skinfold thickness and waist circumference are almost exclusively used.

BMI is calculated using the weight in kilograms divided by height in meters squared and can be reliably used in children over 2 years of age. The normal standards of BMI for children and adolescents vary by age and gender and must be plotted on growth curves. A BMI between the 85th and 95th percentiles defines overweight. A BMI above the 95th percentile defines obesity.

BMI does not distinguish between excess fat, muscle mass, or bone density nor can it be used to define severe obesity, which is defined as a calculated BMI greater than 99th percentile (the 2000 Centers for Disease Control and Prevention growth charts are unable to accurately define and display BMI percentiles beyond the 97th percentile). Although BMI does have its limitations and does not directly measure an individual's body fat, it can be correlated with body fat[1] and is useful and practical as a diagnostic measure in identifying children and adolescents at increased risk of adult-onset obesity.

As a clinician, it is important to recognize the social stigma of overweight and obesity. The term, *fat*, can be associated with concepts of laziness, unattractiveness, and even stupidity. It cannot be stressed enough that care must be taken in the disclosure of these diagnoses to patients and parents. Patients and families may be sensitive to this personal diagnosis and may feel emotions of embarrassment, shame, hopelessness, or even depression by the diagnosis and development of its comorbidities. Some patients and families may even feel judged by their primary provider and team. In addition, providers must be aware that patients and families of different cultures may hold different values regarding weight and body image, which must be taken into account. During these discussions, care must be taken to ascertain patients' and families' explanatory models regarding the diagnosis of overweight or obesity. The explanatory model includes not only the concept of the disease but also the expectations regarding management and outcomes. If differences between the explanatory models of the clinician and the patient/family are not discovered and addressed early on in the therapeutic relationship, the clinical outcome is likely to be poor. Cultural humility must always be the basis of any clinical encounter, because all clinical encounters with patients and families are cross-cultural.

To give a global perspective of the obesity epidemic, more than 50% of the 671 million obese individuals in the world live in 10 countries. As of 2013, the United States of America accounted for 13% of obese people worldwide, with China and India together accounting for 15%. No single country has had any recent significant decline in the rate of obesity.[25]

As discussed previously, in the United States, approximately 17% of children 2 to 19 years old are obese. That amounts to approximately 12.7 million obese children and adolescents. Aside from the ethnic distinctions, prevalence of overweight and obesity in female children and adolescents was directly correlated with the education level of the adult head of the household. Similar findings were not noted in male children.[1]

Multiple studies have shown that vulnerable populations do benefit from public health initiatives to reduce the rate of rise in the obesity epidemic, suggesting this epidemic is controllable with efforts starting with early identification and prevention.

Obesity is a major cause of preventable diseases, such as diabetes, hypertension, cardiovascular disease, sleep apnea, osteoarthritis, cancer, gallbladder disease, and mental health issues. Many of these comorbidities are becoming more prevalent in childhood, particularly among those children in the severe obesity category, who make up 4% to 6% of all youth in the United States.[4]

Assessment

In 2007 an American Academy of Pediatrics Expert Committee developed recommendations for the assessment of child and adolescent overweight and obesity.[26] The latest update of these recommendations was published in October of 2015[27] (**Box 1**).

Following the accurate determination and plotting of BMI/BMI%, the recommendations vary depending on which of the following categories the youth falls into:

1. Healthy weight (BMI 5%–84%)
2. Overweight (BMI 85%–94%)
3. Obesity (BMI $\geq$95%)

For all categories, routine family history, review of symptoms, and physical examination are recommended. For a child/adolescent who is either overweight or obese, an augmented, obesity-specific evaluation is recommended. The augmented evaluation should include inquiry and examination for risk factors associated with overweight/obesity-related conditions that include involvement of dermatologic, endocrine, gastrointestinal, neurologic, orthopedic, and psychological/behavioral health conditions (**Box 2**). Comorbidities identified during the assessment require further work-up, including additional laboratory testing. In 2014, the Children's Hospital Association produced a consensus statement of recommendations describing the management of some comorbidities.[28,29]

TREATMENT
Overview

The American Academy of Pediatrics recommends a 4-stage approach to the management and treatment of patients with overweight and obesity, emphasizing lifestyle changes and age-appropriate dietary counseling (**Table 2**). They recommend starting at the least intensive stage and advancing through the stages based on the response. Counseling should be empowering and supportive and should include the patient and family to positively change behaviors. Weight loss should be limited to 1 lb/mo for obese children 2 to 5 years and 2 lb per week for older children and adolescents.

Nutritional Intervention

Virtually no clinical randomized control trials examining the long-term effects of any specific dietary prescription on BMI or adiposity that control for potentially confounding factors exists. Thus dietary recommendations regarding the treatment of

---

Box 1

Foundations of 2007 American Academy of Pediatrics Expert Committee recommendations for assessment

1. An assessment of eating and activity behaviors of each child/adolescent

2. Provision of preventive counseling (5-2-1-0) for each child/adolescent

3. Determination of weight classification (BMI/BMI%) for each child/adolescent

Box 2
2007 American Academy of Pediatrics Expert Committee recommendations for obese children/adolescents without identified risk factors

1. Support continued healthy lifestyle behaviors.

2. Obtain a nonfasting lipid profile between the ages of 9 to 11 and again at 18 to 21 years.

3. Overweight patients should have a lipid profile at any age.

4. Reassess annually during well-child visit and identify high-risk youth who are crossing 2 percentile lines.

If a child/adolescent is obese or a risk factor(s) is identified, the recommendations include the following:

1. Laboratory tests: fasting glucose, fasting lipid profile, alanine aminotransferase, and aspartate aminotransferase

2. Following the American Diabetes Association and Endocrine Society recommendations using hemoglobin A_{1c}, fasting glucose, or oral glucose tolerance to test for diabetes or prediabetes[30]

3. May obtain nonfasting laboratory tests for patient convenience

4. Determination and timing of follow-up can be based on clinical judgment.

5. The clinical utility of measuring vitamin D and fasting insulin is yet to be determined.

6. At present, there are no guidelines for when to start laboratory testing for obesity.

Table 2
American Academy of Pediatrics 4-stage approach to treatment and management of overweight and obesity

Stage 1: prevention plus	Office-based monthly visits of 15–20 min focusing on realistic behavior changes resulting in weight maintenance or a decrease in BMI velocity. Consider partnering with community services and professionals especially with a dietician. If no improvement in 3–6 mo, consider advancing to stage 2.
Stage 2: structured weight management	Office-based with appropriate training. Similar to stage 1 with more frequent visits (2–4 wk). Emphasis on positive behavior changes including more intense support and structure. Advance to stage 3 without any improvement in 3–6 mo.
Stage 3: comprehensive multidisciplinary intervention	Pediatric weight management clinic staffed by a multidisciplinary team. Weekly or at least every 2–4 wk. Structured behavioral modification with development of short-term diet and physical activity goals. Advance to stage 4 without any improvement in 3–6 mo.
Stage 4: tertiary care intervention	Pediatric weight management center staffed by providers with expertise in treating childhood obesity. Recommended for youth with no improvement in stage 3 who are either ≥95% and significant comorbidities or ≥99%. Intensive diet and activity counseling with consideration of the use of medications and surgery.

childhood obesity must be made from inferences related to the literature on childhood obesity prevention and adult treatment literature. Today, the most common interventions involve the use of balanced macronutrient/low-energy diets. The United States Department of Agriculture MyPlate (**Fig. 1**), which illustrates the 5 food groups that are the building blocks of a healthy diet, and the American Academy of Pediatrics endorsement of the 5-2-1-0 program are excellent starting points for any nutritional counseling:

- Five or more servings of fruits and vegetables a day
- Two hours or less of recreational screen time per day
- One hour or more of daily physical activity
- Zero consumption of sugar sweetened drinks

Behavioral Interventions

Comprehensive behavioral interventions of medium to high intensity have been shown to be effective in reducing BMI among obese or overweight children if provided over a 12-month period. Some evidence is available that these weight reductions can be maintained over an additional 12 months after cessation of the intervention.[31] Specific therapies, including family-based, motivational interviewing and group therapy, continue to demonstrate effectiveness in treating obese children and adolescents, but long-term success without continuing therapy using these interventions is extremely limited.[32–35]

Pharmacotherapy

Medication use is only recommended either after an unsuccessful attempt at weight loss after the adoption of a healthy reduced-calorie diet and an increase in physical activity. Only a single medication (orlistat) has been approved by the US Food and Drug Administration for prescription use in individuals greater than or equal to 12 years of age. This medication reduces the absorption of fats from food and is recommended to be taken with each meal. Cramping, excessive gas, and oily stools

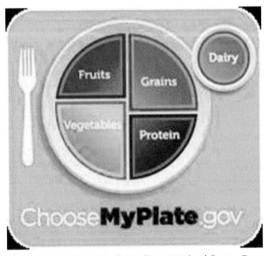

Fig. 1. US Department of Agriculture MyPlate. (*From* United States Department of Agriculture. ChooseMyPlate. Available at: http://www.choosemyplate.gov/. Accessed July 18, 2016.)

are major and frequent side effects and make it difficult to maintain compliance with the medication.[31] Sibutramine, an appetite suppressant that is a nonselective reuptake inhibitor, has been used with pediatric patients but is no longer available for use in the United States.

Limited data exist regarding the use of medication in combination with behavioral interventions. Orlistat was associated with a small (0.85 kg/m^2) weight reduction whereas sibutramine was associated with a moderate (2.6 kg/m^2) weight reduction in obese adolescents while on the medication. At present, there are no studies reporting what happens after cessation of medication.[31]

Metformin is a medication that is considered for use in obese children and adolescents with type 2 diabetes mellitus or prediabetes. Some clinicians are now considering using this medication in treating obese children and adolescents with neither of these conditions. A systematic review of the literature showed a statistically significant but modest reduction in BMI (<5%) when combined with lifestyle interventions over the short term.[36]

The increasing prevalence of nonalcoholic fatty liver disease among children and adolescents has been partially linked to an association with childhood obesity. Lifestyle changes have been recommended as the first-line treatment of this condition. Vitamin E can be considered for those with biopsy-proved nonalcoholic steatohepatitis (NASH) or borderline NASH after failure of lifestyle changes.[37]

Multiple medicines, including lorcaserin, phentermine, topiramate, bupropion, naltrexone, and liraglutide, have been approved by the Food and Drug Administration for use in adults (**Box 3**). All are recommended as an adjunct to lifestyle changes. Only approximately 5% to 10% of additional weight loss on average can be expected from a starting weight but gradual weight gain can be expected with cessation of the medicine.[38]

Bariatric Surgery

Bariatric surgery has become a treatment option for morbidly obese adolescents. As an ancillary study to its observational study of adults undergoing bariatric surgery the National Institute of Diabetes and Digestive and Kidney Diseases created Teen-Longitudinal Assessment of Bariatric Surgery (Teen-LABS) (5 centers in the United States) to serve as a prospective observational cohort study aimed at assessing the clinical, epidemiologic, and behavioral parameters in a select population of bariatric surgical (**Box 4**) patients.[39]

Box 3
Pharmacotherapy for overweight and obesity

- Sibutramine
- Orlistat
- Metformin
- Vitamin E (tocopherol)
- Lorcaserin
- Topiramate
- Bupropion
- Naltrexone
- Liraglutide

> **Box 4**
> **Criteria for inclusion in the National Institute of Diabetes and Digestive and Kidney Diseases Teen-LABS study**
>
> - Failed more than 6 months of organized attempts at weight management
> - Have attained or nearly attained physiologic maturity
> - Greater than 50 BMI or greater than 40 BMI with an associated severe comorbidity (ie, sleep apnea, diabetes, or hypertension)
> - Demonstrate commitment to comprehensive medical and psychological evaluations both before and after surgery
> - Agree to avoid pregnancy for at least 1 year
> - Be capable and willing to adhere to nutritional guidelines postoperatively
> - Provide informed consent
> - Demonstrate decisional capacity
> - Have a supportive family environment

Analysis of the data 3 years after surgery (Roux-en-Y gastric bypass or sleeve gastrectomy in 242 adolescents) showed significant improvements in weight-related quality of life, cardiometabolic health, and weight with an associated manageable low incidence of surgical complications and specific micronutrient deficiencies.[40] Additional studies support these findings of significant short-term (<3 years) weight loss, quality-of-life improvement, and safety.

School-Based/Community/Hospital

Multiple initiatives have been proposed or implemented to increase the involvement of schools and communities in combating the epidemic of childhood obesity. Many of the programs are adopted with good intentions but little analysis exists of the programs, especially in children and adolescents.

A study completed in California found that school-based BMI screening and parent notification were not associated with BMI changes.[41] In 2003, Arkansas was one of the first states that required that all children attending public schools be screened for their BMI and the information sent home. In 2007 the state altered the legislation allowing for parental opt-out and alternate-year collection of BMI. A secondary analysis of Youth Risk Behavior Surveys completed in 2005, 2007, and 2009 demonstrated that continued exposure of 11th and 12th graders to BMI screening and reporting was not associated with adolescent' health outcomes.[42]

The Federal Healthy, Hunger-Free Kids Act passed in 2012 brought about the first change for school meals in 15 years. The changes aligned school lunches with the dietary guidelines of 2010. A great deal of controversy arose involving the implementation of these requirements specifically related to costs, possible decrease in the number of participants in the school lunch program, and possible increased food waste. A recent publication reported that in a specific school district the new meal standards effectively changed the quality of foods selected by both middle and high school students in an urban school district.[43]

A great deal of interest is now being placed on introducing warning labels on sugar-sweetened beverages (SSBs). A recent study demonstrated that warning labels can alter a parent's selection of an SSB, use of coupons for an SSB, and the intent to purchase future SSBs for children between the ages of 6 and 10 years. No differences in parental behaviors were noted in the message imparted on the warning label.[44]

Obese children and adolescents attending a summer residential camp exclusively designed for this population have been shown to lose a significant amount of weight. Unfortunately most regain the weight on return to home. Treatment of severely obese children and adolescents in an in-patient facility was shown superior to treatment in an ambulatory setting but weight loss was not sustained on long-term follow-up.[45]

Social Media

Research involving use of technology platforms that are already integrated into the lives of adolescents and young adults are rapidly beginning to appear in the obesity-related literature. Privacy barriers still exist to the provision of many interventions directly to adolescents less than 18 years of age. Research completed with young adults, however, is beginning to highlight some positive results, including efficacy and acceptability.[46,47]

Financing

Recently the authors completed a study assessing reimbursement for services provided by a nutritionist and a physician in a referral-based weight management clinic (part time over a 6-month period). They exclusively billed the *International Classification of Diseases, Ninth Revision*, code for obesity (278.00) and either the *Current Procedural Terminology* code of 99,204 (new) or 99,213 (follow-up) for physician services. No bill was submitted for nutrition services; 76 individual adolescents (34 new and 42 follow-up) were included in the study that made a total of 149 visits. There were 29 individual insurance carriers. Total collections were 24.12% ($14,646.67) of the total billings. The estimated cost for staffing a pediatric weight management center with an interdisciplinary team would be approximately $750,000. At present, reimbursement to sustain a pediatric weight management center with an interdisciplinary team seems inadequate.[48]

SUMMARY

Health is not only the absence of disease. It is also happiness, peace of mind, and the ability to fulfill full potential in life. As children continue to lose their health to overweight and obesity, the United States and other nations will suffer the loss of economic, educational, scientific, and creative contributions from able-bodied and sound-minded adults, all this while the cost of health care continues to rise and federal reserves buckle under the added weight of caring for so many children and adults suffering from devastating comorbidities.

Further research is critically needed in the areas of prevention and treatment of children, specifically, as is advocacy to push for funding of community resources in low-income areas, and protect physical education programs in schools. Pediatric health care providers must support the efforts of medical academies and societies and initiate efforts where they are lacking. Internists and adult-medicine specialists must join the efforts of pediatricians in pushing for improved resources for children to address adult obesity and its consequences. Finally, the topics of childhood overweight and obesity as well as cross-cultural communication and methods, such as motivational interviewing, must be increased in medical school curricula and continuing education for providers.

REFERENCES

1. Centers for Disease Control and Prevention. Childhood Overweight and Obesity. Available at: http://www.cdc.gov/obesity/childhood/index.html.
2. The National health and nutrition examination survey, 2009-2010. Available at: https://wwwn.cdc.gov/Nchs/Nhanes/Search/Nhanes09_10.aspx.
3. Ogden CL, Carroll MD, Kit BK, et al. Prevalence of childhood and adult obesity in the United States, 2011-2012. JAMA 2014;311(8):806–14.
4. Kelly AS, Barlow SE, Rao G, et al. Severe obesity in children and adolescents: identification, associated health risks, and treatment approaches: a scientific statement from the American Heart Association. Circulation 2013;128:1689–712.
5. Expert Panel on Integrated Guidelines for Cardiovascular Health and Risk Reduction in Children and Adolescents, National Heart, Lung, and Blood Institute. Expert panel on integrated guidelines for cardiovascular health and risk reduction in children and adolescents: summary report. Pediatrics 2011;128:S213–56.
6. Hansen ML, Gunn PW, Kaelber DC. Underdiagnosis of hypertension in children and adolescents. JAMA 2007;298:874–9.
7. Gidding SS, Nehgme R, Heise C, et al. Severe obesity associated with cardiovascular deconditioning, high prevalence of cardiovascular risk factors, diabetes mellitus/hyperinsulinemia, and respiratory compromise. J Pediatr 2004;144(6):766–9.
8. Friend A, Craig L, Turner S. The prevalence of metabolic syndrome in children: a systematic review of the literature. Metab Syndr Relat Disord 2013;11(2):71–80.
9. Pettitt DJ, Talton J, Dabelea D, et al. Prevalence of diabetes in U.S. youth in 2009: the SEARCH for diabetes in youth study. Diabetes Care 2014;37(2):402–8.
10. Sinha R, Fisch G, Teague B, et al. Prevalence of impaired glucose tolerance among children and adolescents with marked obesity. N Engl J Med 2002;346:802–10.
11. Novais EN, Millis MB. Slipped capital femoral epiphysis: prevalence, pathogenesis, and natural history. Clin Orthop Relat Res 2012;470:3432–8.
12. Small L, Aplasca A. Child obesity and mental health: a complex interaction. Child Adolesc Psychiatr Clin N Am 2016;25(2):269–82.
13. Freedman DS, Mei Z, Srinivasan SR, et al. Cardiovascular risk factors and excess adiposity among overweight children and adolescents: the bogalusa heart study. J Pediatr 2007;150(1):12–7.e2.
14. Chen D, Thomsen MR, Nayga RM. Persistent disparities in obesity risk among public schoolchildren from childhood through adolescence. Prev Med 2016;89:207–10.
15. Subica AM, Grills CT, Douglas JA, et al. Communities of color creating healthy environments to combat childhood obesity. Am J Public Health 2016;106(1):79–86.
16. Watson KB, Harris CD, Carlson SA, et al. Disparities in adolescents' residence in neighborhoods supportive of physical activity - United States, 2011-2012. MMWR Morb Mortal Wkly Rep 2016;65(23):598–601.
17. Woo Baidal JA, Locks LM, Cheng ER, et al. Risk factors for childhood obesity in the first 1,000 days: a systematic review. Am J Prev Med 2016;50(6):761–79.
18. Mech P, Hooley M, Skouteris H, et al. Parent-related mechanisms underlying the social gradient of childhood overweight and obesity: a systematic review. Child Care Health Dev 2016. http://dx.doi.org/10.1111/cch.12356.
19. Pei Z, Flexeder C, Fuertes E, et al. Mother's body mass index and food intake in school-aged children: results of the GINIplus and the LISAplus studies. Eur J Clin Nutr 2014;68(8):898–906.

20. Gibbs BG, Forste R. Socioeconomic status, infant feeding practices and early childhood obesity. Pediatr Obes 2014;9:135–46.

21. Bouchard C, Tremblay A, Despres JP, et al. The response to long-term overfeeding in identical twins. N Engl J Med 1990;322:1477–82.

22. Turta O, Rautava S. Antibiotics, obesity, and the link to microbes – what are we doing to our children? BMC Med 2016;14:57.

23. Scott FI, Horton DB. Administration of antibiotics to children before age 2 years increases risk for childhood obesity. Gastroenterology 2016;151:120–9.

24. Parrino C, Vinciguerra F, La Spina N. Influence of early-life and parental factors on childhood overweight and obesity. J Endocrinol Invest 2016. [Epub ahead of print].

25. Krebs NF, Himes JH, Jacobson D, et al. Assessment of child and adolesent overweight and obesity. Pediatrics 2007;120:S193–228.

26. Barlow S, Expert Committee. Expert committee recommendations regarding prevention, assessment, and treatment of child and adolescent overweight and obesity. Summary report. Pediatrics 2007;120(4):S164–92.

27. American Academy of Pediatrics Institute for healthy childhood weight. Algorithm for the assessment and management of childhood obesity in patients 2 years and older. American Academy of Pediatrics Institute for Healthy Childhood Weight. Available at: https://ihcw.aap.org/Documents/Assessment%20and%20Management%20of%20Childhood%20Obesity%20Algorithm_v1015.pdf

28. Estrada E, Eneli I, Hampl S. Children's Hospital Association consensus statements for comorbidities of childhood obesity. Child Obes 2014;10(4):304–17.

29. Haemer MA, Grow HM, Fernandez C, et al. Addressing prediabetes in childhood obesity treatment programs: Support from research and current practice. Child Obes 2014;10(4):292–303.

30. American Diabetes Association. Classification and diagnosis of diabetes. Sec.2. Standards of medical care in diabetes- 2015. Diabetes Care 2015;38(Suppl 1): S8–16.

31. Whitlock EP, O'Connor EA, Williams SB, et al. Effectiveness of weight management interventions in children: a targeted systematic review for the USPSTF. Pediatrics 2010;125:e396–418.

32. Taylor RW, Cox A, Knight L, et al. A tailored family-based obesity intervention: a randomized trial. Pediatrics 2015;136(2):281–9.

33. Broccoli S, Davoli AM, Bonvicini L, et al. Motivational interviewing to treat overweight children: 24-month follow-up of a randomized controlled trial. Pediatrics 2016;137(1):1–10.

34. Resnicow K, Mcmaster F, Bocian A, et al. Motivational interviewing and dietary counseling for obesity in primary care: an RCT. Pediatrics 2015;135(4):649–57.

35. Panzer BM, Dhuper S. Designing a group therapy program for coping with childhood weight bias. Soc Work 2014;59(2):141–7.

36. McDonagh MS, Selph S, Ozpinar A, et al. Systematic review of the benefits and risks of metformin in treating obesity in children aged 18 years and younger. JAMA Pediatr 2014;168(2):178–84.

37. Mitchel EB, Lavine JE. Review article: the management of pediatric nonalcoholic fatty liver disease. Aliment Pharmacol Ther 2014;40:1155–70.

38. Apovian CM, Aronne LJ, Bessesen DH, et al. Pharmacological management of obesity: an Endocrine Society clinical practice guideline. J Clin Endocrinol Metab 2015;100(2):342–62.

39. Inge TH, Zeller M, Harmon C, et al. Teen-longitudinal assessment of bariatric surgery: methodological features of the first prospective multicenter study of adolescent bariatric surgery. J Pediatr Surg 2007;42:1969–71.

40. Inge TH, Courcoulas AP, Jenkins T, et al. Weight loss and health status 3 years after bariatric surgery in adolescents. N Engl J Med 2016;374(2):113–23.

41. Madsen KA. School-based body mass index screening and parent notification: a statewide natural experiment. Arch Pediatr Adolesc Med 2011;165:987–92.

42. Gee KA. School-based body mass index screening and parental notification in late adolescence: Evidence from Arkansas Act 1220. J Adolesc Health 2015; 57:270–6.

43. Johnson DB, Podrabsky M, Rocha A, et al. Effect of the Healthy Hunger-Free Kids Act on the nutritional quality of meals selected by students and school lunch participationrates. JAMA Pediatr 2016;170(1):e153918.

44. Roberto CA, Wong D, Musicus A, et al. The influence of sugar-sweetened beverage health warning labels on parents' choices. Pediatrics 2016;137(2): e20153185.

45. van der Baan-Slootweg O, Benninga MA, Beelan A, et al. Inpatient treatment of children and adolescents with severe obesity in the Netherlands: a randomized clinical trial. JAMA Pediatr 2014;168(9):807–14.

46. Napolitano M, Hayes S, Bennett GG, et al. Using facebook and text messaging to deliver a weight loss program to college students. Obesity (Silver Spring) 2013; 21(1):25–31.

47. Hingle M, Nichter M, Medeiros M, et al. Texting for health; the use of participatory methods to develop healthy lifestyle messages for teens. J Nutr Educ Behav 2013;45(1):12–9.

48. Feinstein RA, DiFiglia-Peck S, Wahab Y. Financing a weight management program for overweight/obese adolescents. Baltimore (MD): Pediatric Academic Society; 2016.

Index

Note: Page numbers of article titles are in **boldface** type.

Gastroenterol Clin N Am 45 (2016) 729–736
http://dx.doi.org/10.1016/S0889-8553(16)30100-5
0889-8553/16

UNITED STATES POSTAL SERVICE® Statement of Ownership, Management, and Circulation (All Periodicals Publications Except Requester Publications)

1. Publication Title	2. Publication Number	3. Filing Date
GASTROENTEROLOGY CLINICS OF NORTH AMERICA	000 – 279	9/18/16

4. Issue Frequency	5. Number of Issues Published Annually	6. Annual Subscription Price
MAR, JUN, SEP, DEC	4	$305.00

7. Complete Mailing Address of Known Office of Publication (Not printer) (Street, city, county, state, and ZIP+4®)

ELSEVIER INC.
360 PARK AVENUE SOUTH
NEW YORK, NY 10010-1710

Contact Person
STEPHEN R. BUSHING

Telephone (Include area code)
215-239-3688

8. Complete Mailing Address of Headquarters or General Business Office of Publisher (Not printer)

ELSEVIER INC.
360 PARK AVENUE SOUTH
NEW YORK, NY 10010-1710

9. Full Names and Complete Mailing Addresses of Publisher, Editor, and Managing Editor (Do not leave blank)

Publisher (Name and complete mailing address)

ADRIANNE BRIGIDO, ELSEVIER INC.
1600 JOHN F KENNEDY BLVD. SUITE 1800
PHILADELPHIA, PA 19103-2899

Editor (Name and complete mailing address)

KERRY HOLLAND, ELSEVIER INC.
1600 JOHN F KENNEDY BLVD. SUITE 1800
PHILADELPHIA, PA 19103-2899

Managing Editor (Name and complete mailing address)

PATRICK MANLEY, ELSEVIER INC.
1600 JOHN F KENNEDY BLVD. SUITE 1800
PHILADELPHIA, PA 19103-2899

10. Owner (Do not leave blank. If the publication is owned by a corporation, give the name and address of the corporation immediately followed by the names and addresses of all stockholders owning or holding 1 percent or more of the total amount of stock. If not owned by a corporation, give the names and addresses of the individual owners. If owned by a partnership or other unincorporated firm, give its name and address as well as those of each individual owner. If the publication is published by a nonprofit organization, give its name and address.)

Full Name	Complete Mailing Address
WHOLLY OWNED SUBSIDIARY OF REED/ELSEVIER US HOLDINGS	1600 JOHN F KENNEDY BLVD. SUITE 1800 PHILADELPHIA, PA 19103-2899

11. Known Bondholders, Mortgagees, and Other Security Holders Owning or Holding 1 Percent or More of Total Amount of Bonds, Mortgages, or Other Securities. If none, check box ☐ None

Full Name	Complete Mailing Address
N/A	

12. Tax Status (For completion by nonprofit organizations authorized to mail at nonprofit rates) (Check one)
The purpose, function, and nonprofit status of this organization and the exempt status for federal income tax purposes:
☐ Has Not Changed During Preceding 12 Months
☐ Has Changed During Preceding 12 Months (Publisher must submit explanation of change with this statement)

13. Publication Title
GASTROENTEROLOGY CLINICS OF NORTH AMERICA

14. Issue Date for Circulation Data Below
JUNE 2016

15. Extent and Nature of Circulation		Average No. Copies Each Issue During Preceding 12 Months	No. Copies of Single Issue Published Nearest to Filing Date
a. Total Number of Copies (Net press run)		492	506
b. Paid Circulation (By Mail and Outside the Mail)	(1) Mailed Outside-County Paid Subscriptions Stated on PS Form 3541 (Include paid distribution above nominal rate, advertiser's proof copies, and exchange copies)	136	153
	(2) Mailed In-County Paid Subscriptions Stated on PS Form 3541 (Include paid distribution above nominal rate, advertiser's proof copies, and exchange copies)	0	0
	(3) Paid Distribution Outside the Mails Including Sales Through Dealers and Carriers, Street Vendors, Counter Sales, and Other Paid Distribution Outside USPS®	109	116
	(4) Paid Distribution by Other Classes of Mail Through the USPS (e.g., First-Class Mail®)	0	0
c. Total Paid Distribution [Sum of 15b (1), (2), (3), and (4)]		245	269
d. Free or Nominal Rate Distribution (By Mail and Outside the Mail)	(1) Free or Nominal Rate Outside-County Copies included on PS Form 3541	68	87
	(2) Free or Nominal Rate In-County Copies included on PS Form 3541	0	0
	(3) Free or Nominal Rate Copies Mailed at Other Classes Through the USPS (e.g., First-Class Mail)	0	0
	(4) Free or Nominal Rate Distribution Outside the Mail (Carriers or other means)	0	0
e. Total Free or Nominal Rate Distribution (Sum of 15d (1), (2), (3) and (4))		68	87
f. Total Distribution (Sum of 15c and 15e)		313	356
g. Copies not Distributed (See Instructions to Publishers #4 (page #3))		179	150
h. Total (Sum of 15f and g)		492	506
i. Percent Paid (15c divided by 15f times 100)		78%	76%

* If you are claiming electronic copies, go to line 16 on page 3. If you are not claiming electronic copies, skip to line 17 on page 3.

16. Electronic Copy Circulation	Average No. Copies Each Issue During Preceding 12 Months	No. Copies of Single Issue Published Nearest to Filing Date
a. Paid Electronic Copies ▶	0	0
b. Total Paid Print Copies (Line 15c) + Paid Electronic Copies (Line 16a) ▶	245	269
c. Total Print Distribution (Line 15f) + Paid Electronic Copies (Line 16a) ▶	313	356
d. Percent Paid (Both Print & Electronic Copies) (16b divided by 16c × 100) ▶	78%	76%

☒ I certify that 50% of all my distributed copies (electronic and print) are paid above a nominal price.

17. Publication of Statement of Ownership
☒ If the publication is a general publication, publication of this statement is required. Will be printed in the DECEMBER 2016 issue of this publication.
☐ Publication not required.

18. Signature and Title of Editor, Publisher, Business Manager, or Owner

STEPHEN R. BUSHING - INVENTORY DISTRIBUTION CONTROL MANAGER

Date 9/18/16

I certify that all information furnished on this form is true and complete. I understand that anyone who furnishes false or misleading information on this form or who omits material or information requested on the form may be subject to criminal sanctions (including fines and imprisonment) and/or civil sanctions (including civil penalties).

PS Form 3526, July 2014 (Page 3 of 4)   PRIVACY NOTICE: See our privacy policy on www.usps.com

PS Form 3526, July 2014 [Page 1 of 4] (see instructions page 4)]   PSN 7530-01-000-9931   PRIVACY NOTICE: See our privacy policy on www.usps.com

Moving?

Make sure your subscription moves with you!

To notify us of your new address, find your **Clinics Account Number** (located on your mailing label above your name), and contact customer service at:

Email: journalscustomerservice-usa@elsevier.com

800-654-2452 (subscribers in the U.S. & Canada)
314-447-8871 (subscribers outside of the U.S. & Canada)

Fax number: 314-447-8029

Elsevier Health Sciences Division
Subscription Customer Service
3251 Riverport Lane
Maryland Heights, MO 63043

*To ensure uninterrupted delivery of your subscription, please notify us at least 4 weeks in advance of move.

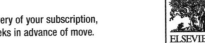

Printed and bound by CPI Group (UK) Ltd, Croydon, CR0 4YY

07/10/2024

01040502-0016